Diminishing Corruptive Practices in the Public Hospital System of Cameroon:
A Qualitative Multiple Case Study

Dr. Foleng M. Ndofor, Ph.D

Langaa Research & Publishing CIG
Mankon, Bamenda

Publisher

Langaa RPCIG
Langaa Research & Publishing Common Initiative Group
P.O. Box 902 Mankon
Bamenda
North West Region
Cameroon
Langaagrp@gmail.com
www.langaa-rpcig.net

Distributed in and outside N. America by African Books Collective
orders@africanbookscollective.com
www.africanbookscollective.com

ISBN-10: 9956-550-67-1

ISBN-13: 978-9956-550-67-8

© Dr. Foleng M. Ndofor, Ph.D 2019

Table of Contents

List of Tables and Figures

Tables

Figures

Abstract

Corrupt business and management practices exist at all levels within the public hospital system (PHS) in Cameroon and are of increasing concern among the polity as the perceptions of key stakeholders who work within the system has not been examined for helping to diminish it. Specifically, these practices are affecting the well-being of Cameroonians and its socioeconomic development. The problem that needed to be addressed was the corrupt business and management practices that continue to lead to increased monetary cost to individuals and delays in seeking preventative care within the PHS. The purpose of this qualitative, multiple case study was to provide further understanding of how to diminish corrupt business and management practices that continue to lead to increased monetary cost to individuals and delays in seeking preventative care within the PHS. Stakeholder theory provided a starting point for understanding and explaining the perceptions of stakeholders about corruption within the context of agency governance. Semi-structured, open-ended telephone interviews were conducted with nine participants (three nurses, three nurse managers, and three physicians) who worked in various administrative realms within a regional hospital in Cameroon. Each interview was recorded, transcript verbatim, and analyzed using thematic deductive analysis. The results indicated that staff/client influence rather than only motivation was a rationale for stakeholder engagement in accepting bribes. A key finding of the study was the revelation of two other forms of corruption: (a) diversion in which physicians keeps drugs in their office for sale to patients and (b) extortion in which staff members condition type of service provided to level of patronage received. As a measure for diminishing corruption, it was revealed that a strong anti-corruption body that is legally grounded be installed in all departments; however, research on the requirements for setting up anti-corrupt bodies that are anchored in the legal system is lacking in current research. Additional research is recommended for investigating the requirements for setting up such anti-corruption bodies. Such research might qualitatively be designed to include other public hospitals facing similar issues with corruption and using research questions that asks stakeholder perceptions of ways in designing and implementing it.

Acknowledgements

I owe my deepest gratitude to Prof. Daniel Pitchford, who worked tirelessly to make this work possible. His expertise, high standards, and advice were critical in realizing this book. I am equally grateful to Dr. Tippins, Dr. Abigail Scheg, and Dr. Sharon Kimmel for their suggestions, feedbacks, and encouragements in realizing this project. Most important of all is the support of my family: my wife Virgie and daughter Abong who sacrificed their personal time and attention to allow me to write. My profound gratitude also goes to my wonderful parents: Mr. Clement Ndofor (late) and Mrs. Winifred Ndofor. The sacrifices you both made in raising me in a caring home cannot be repaid with monetary value. Finally, I like to extend my deepest appreciation to my friends, brothers, and sisters with their families: Mr. & Mrs. Stephen Ndofor, Mr. & Mrs. Denis Ndebum, Mr. Norbert & Family, Mr. & Mrs. Nico Ndofor, Miss. Judith Ndofor (late), Mami Anastasia & Family, Mr. & Mrs. Julian Ndofor, and Vernita Ndofor. Your steadfast support, prayers, and best wishes during this process was uplifting and encouraging. Thank you all!

Chapter 1

Introduction

Corrupt business and management practices exist at all levels within the public hospital system (PHS) in Cameroon and are of increasing concern among the polity as the perceptions of stakeholders (nurse managers, nurses, and physicians) who work within the system has not been examined for helping to diminish it (Kankeu et al., 2016; Kankeu & Ventelou, 2016; Tinyami et al., 2015; Yamb & Bayemi, 2017). In particular, these practices are affecting the healthcare outcomes of Cameroonians and the socioeconomic development of the country. Recently, a study on the state of corruption within the PHS, revealed that about 31% of individuals who visited or seek treatment at a public hospital had paid a bribe or "informal" payment to receive better care, avoid being in queues, and see a doctor compared to 24% in 2010 (Kankeu et al., 2016; Yamb & Bayemi, 2017). It also showed that about 61% of the public found the system to be very corrupt. The PHS plays a vital role in the well-being of the polity because of its core mission of preventing, improving and delivering better healthcare services (Kankeu et al., 2016; Kankeu & Ventelou, 2016; Njong & Ngantcha, 2013; Yamb & Bayemi, 2017).

The PHS consists of several public entities, organizations and institutions that fall under the management of the Ministry of Public Health (MoPH), including the national teaching and university hospital, regional, divisional, and sub-divisional or rural hospitals and pharmacies (Molem-Christopher et al., 2017; Tinyami, et al., 2015). Within the hospital system, the MoPH oversees the management of all public healthcare related services. The PHS through its regional hospitals in all 10 Regions of the country accounts for most of the healthcare services that are provided to the public (Kankeu & Ventelou, 2016). Funding for the PHS comes primarily from the government, which spends about 4.1% of its gross domestic product GDP or $61 per capital (Kankeu & Ventelou, 2016). Other funding sources come from international bodies such as the World Health Organization (WHO), the European Union (EU), the World Bank (WB), and the public (Kankeu & Ventelou, 2016). The top management is among the areas that corrupt business and management practices is existing.

Within the top management charged with regulating and coordinating health policies and systems, including reference and teaching hospitals, corruption exists in the form of bribes or "informal" payments paid to officials and employees (Kankeu et al., 2016; Njong & Ngantcha, 2013; Osifo, 2014). Family members and patients make these payments themselves as a condition for accessing and receiving better treatment and care services at in-patient facilities, as well as out-patient facilities at reference and teaching hospital (Kankeu et al., 2016; Yamb & Bayemi, 2017). In addition, corruption occurs in the theft and sale of drugs like anti-retroviral that has been donated or purchased by the government which are supposed to be free to patients seeking treatments for the Human Immune Virus and Acquired Immune Deficiency Syndrome (HIV/AIDS; Kankeu et al., 2017; Stearns et al., 2017; Yamb & Bayemi, 2017).

Because of this, it has resulted in extra monetary cost to individuals, as well as their families and delays in seeking medical treatment (Jakubowski et al., 2017; Yamb & Bayemi, 2017). Delays in seeking medical treatment has led to an increase in the number of people especially young adults that are living with HIV/AIDS and early death of children under the age of five dying of preventable illness like malaria (Kankeu & Ventelou, 2016; Hajizadeh, Sia, Heymann & Nandi, 2014; Tinyami et al.,

2

2015). The administration of the PHS is another area where corruption is occurring.

Within the administration of the PHS, consisting of secretary generals, directors and regional delegates who are responsible for appointing and delegating responsibilities to personnel corruption exists in bribes paid by medical doctors and staff members to superiors to avoid transfers to rural areas and maintaining "nice" positions (Yamb & Bayemi, 2017, p. 98). Such practices which have resulted to an uneven distribution of qualified healthcare personnel especially in rural areas, in the ratio of 1.3 to 1,000 has led to a high rate of neonatal deaths of 95 per 1,000 live births (Montoya et al., 2014; Tinyami et al., 2015). Furthermore, corrupt business practices occur in the abuse of delegated authority by officials in appointing and promoting family and clan members in senior positions without consideration for other prospective applicants irrespective of agency policies against such practices. In addition, corruption occurs in the demands of "informal" monetary payments paid by students and their parents as a condition for admission into the sole medical training college (Okafor et al., 2014; Yamb & Bayemi, 2017).

Such practices deny other qualified potential applicants equal opportunities and results in inefficiencies in the coordination of HIV/AIDS programs and lack of preventive strategies in combatting infectious diseases like cholera and malaria. Because of this, it has led to recent increases in the prevalence of these diseases among children and young adults (Djouma, Ateudjieu, Ram, Debes & Sack, 2016; Okafor et al., 2014; Yamb & Bayemi, 2017). The management of healthcare services is another level within the PHS where corruption is occurring.

Within the periphery or bottom administration level, which consists of frontline employees responsible for day-to-day operations including, infant immunization programs, maternal

3

outreach programs and preventive illness programs at regional and sub-regional hospitals and clinics corruption exists in unjustified and unexplained tardiness and absence of employees and some officials during normal business hours, while working a second job as managers or directors remain silent (Molem-Christopher et al., 2017; Ongolo-Zogo et al., 2014; Yamb & Bayemi, 2017). Because of this, it has affected the ability of the PHS to efficiently manage its core mission of improving and delivering better healthcare services to the public leading to longer wait times in queues to see a doctor, delays in responding to patient calls or requests and increase in nurse and physician workload (Kankeu et al., 2016; Kankeu & Ventelou, 2016; Njong & Ngantcha, 2013; Yamb & Bayemi, 2017).

Problem of the Study

The problem that needed to be addressed was the corrupt business and management practices that continue to lead to increased monetary cost to individuals and delays in seeking preventative care within the PHS (Kankeu et al., 2016; Tinyami et al., 2016; Yamb & Bayemi, 2017). In particular, studies (Kankeu et al., 2016; Osifo, 2014; Njong & Ngantcha, 2013; Tinyami et al., 2016; Yamb & Bayemi, 2017) have revealed that corrupt business and management practices within the PHS exist in the form of bribes or "informal" payments that are paid to officials and employees. Patients and their families make these payments themselves as a condition for accessing and receiving better treatment and care services at in-patient, as well as out-patient facilities at reference, regional and sub-regional hospitals (Kankeu et al., 2016; Yamb & Bayemi, 2017).

Additionally, corruption occurs in the theft and sale of hospital supplies such as mosquito nets for preventing malaria infection and drugs used in treating patients who are taking treatment for (HIV/AIDS; Kankeu et al., 2017; Stearns et al.,

2017; Yamb & Bayemi, 2017). Such corrupt business and management practices lead to monetary cost to individuals and delays in seeking preventive medical care (Jakubowski et al., 2017; Yamb & Bayemi, 2017). Delays in seeking medical care have led to an increase in the number of people especially young adults that are living with HIV/AIDS (Kankeu & Ventelou, 2016; Hajizadeh et al., 2014). Without an investigation into the high prevalence of young adults living with HIV/AIDS, low life expectancy and high infant death rates it may continue to occur and affect the well-being of the public (Kankeu et al., 2016; Njong & Ngantcha, 2013; Osifo, 2014; Yamb & Bayemi, 2016; Yamb & Bayemi, 2017).

Purpose of the Study

The purpose of this qualitative, multiple case study was to provide further understanding of how to diminish corrupt business and management practices that continue to lead to increased monetary cost to individuals and delays in seeking preventative care within the PHS (Kankeu et al., 2016; Njong & Ngantcha, 2013; Yamb & Bayemi, 2017). As such, a multiple case study design was used for its appropriateness in investigating the relevant stakeholders' perceptions of the corrupt business and management practices and measures in diminishing it, something which would be hard to achieve using an experiment in a controlled setting (Yin, 2009).

Semi-structured, open-ended interviews were conducted (with three nurse managers, three nurses and three physicians) at a regional hospital in the Northwest region of Cameroon (Yin, 2009). The interview questions were field-tested based at least on three expert reviews of hospital directors of public health in the PHS ensuring dependability and credibility of the interview questions with the research questions (Kvale, 2008). For a multiple case study, Yin (2013a) suggests a range of 6-10

5

interviews, with six being the lowest number of interviews needed to achieve saturation. If saturation was not met recruitment would have continued to meet saturation requirement (Yin, 2009). For this study, a total of nine participants (three nurse managers, three nurses and three physicians) who work in a specific realm within the PHS in the Northwest region of Cameroon was interviewed (Kvale, 1996). The data was analyzed using a deductive thematic analysis. A deductive thematic analysis is a qualitative method in identifying similar patterns of meaning within a data set (Braun & Clarke, 2017). Participants were recruited from a regional hospital directory in the Northwest region and using a convenience and purposive sampling process.

Conceptual Framework

This study was guided by the stakeholder theoretical framework (Freeman, 1984; Harrison, et al. 2015; Hasnas, 2013). The use of stakeholder theory in understanding and explaining the behaviors and the perceptions of stakeholders within the context of agency governance has been well documented (Freeman, 1984; Harrison, et al., 2015; Hasnas, 2013; Tantalo & Priem, 2014). Stakeholder theory is an agency management theory that was conceptualized and developed by Milton Freeman in 1984 (Freeman, 1984; Tantalo & Priem, 2014). Freeman (1984) defined a stakeholder as an individual or group who can impact the management of agency processes. Thus, the stakeholders of the PHS includes: nurses, officials (nurse managers), physicians, Ministry of Public Health (MoPH), regional and sub-regional in-patient and out-patient hospitals, pharmacies, the public and related inter-agencies (Freeman & Phillips, 2002; Harrison et al., 2015).

Freeman's initial conceptualization of stakeholder theory was a normative effort in analyzing stakeholder behaviors and perceptions within the context of agency governance (Freeman, 1984). Freeman's (1984) initial assumption and the key argument of stakeholder theory is that the success of organizations is dependent upon how effective managers can balance the interests of all its stakeholders while developing and maintaining effective relationships in a manner that increases the long-term value of all stakeholders (Harrison et al., 2015; Tantalo & Priem, 2014). As such, having a profound understanding of stakeholder perceptions is central in shaping and cultivating better business practices (Freeman, 2002; Tantalo & Priem, 2014).

Stakeholder theory guided this study by serving as a conceptual framework in revealing what is unknown about the perceptions of nurse managers, nurses and physicians' interest in corrupt business and management practices, rationale or justification for other corruption and associated problems in diminishing these corrupt practices (Freeman, 2002; Harrison et al., 2015; Hasnas, 2013). Theoretically, because key stakeholders (nurse managers, nurses, physicians) who work or are duly qualified to work within each specific agency in the PHS have the best insights of corrupt business and management practices within each specific agency, a direct inquiry of key stakeholders' perceptions was the best approach in diminishing such practices (Yamb & Bayemi, 2017; Yin, 2009). Practically, the resultant contributions of nurse managers, nurses and physicians perceptions of corrupt business and management practices, including interests in corruption, rationale or justification for corruption and problems associated with diminishing such practices may inform understanding through which top management (Minister of Public Health, regional and sub-regional delegates) may use in developing and enhancing best business and management practices, including policies, procedures and regulations in diminishing all forms of corrupt practices (Freeman, 2002; Harrison et al., 2015; Yamb & Bayemi, 2017).

7

This study contributed to stakeholder theory by determining the relevant perceptions and understandings of a diverse set of key stakeholders' (nurse managers, nurses and physicians) interest in corrupt business and management practices, justification for corrupt practices and problems in diminishing such practices (Freeman, 1984; Freeman, 2002). As top management in the PHS, as well as nurse managers apply the resulting findings of stakeholder perceptions as a foundation for managerial strategy, the likelihood of corrupt business and management practices to occur will diminish (Tormusa & Idom, 2016; Yamb & Bayemi, 201).

Research Questions

The following research questions were used to obtain data for this study:

RQ1: How do stakeholders perceive corrupt business and management practices of bribery in receiving better care at in-patient facilities, unjustified absence and tardiness while being paid, maintaining a "nice" position and promoting and hiring family members to exist in the PHS of Cameroon?

RQ1a: How do stakeholders perceive other corrupt business and management practices that may exist in the PHS of Cameroon?

RQ2: How do stakeholders perceive ways to diminish and improve the business and management practices that exist in the PHS of Cameroon?

Significance of the Study

This study is beneficial in several areas such as (a) identifying and implementing policies design to enhance efficiency in delivering better healthcare services at in-patient and outpatient facilities in reference, regional and sub-regional hospitals, (b)

8

implementing regulations and procedures design to enhance transparency in the selection process, including hiring, promoting and transferring and (c) adopting policies and initiatives design to enhance attendance and work rules, including absenteeism and tardiness (Asongu, 2013; Fry, 2016; Osifo, 2014).

Additionally, the elicited insights of stakeholders might shed more light of potential risk factors that may occur in engendering corrupt business and management practices within the PHS resulting in the implementation of initiatives in identifying and mitigating such potential risks (Fry, 2016; Tormusa & Idom, 2016).

Region. A region is an official name for an administrative area in Cameroon. It is similar to a State in the United States or a Province of Canada. There are 10 regions in Cameroon (Markham & Fonjong, 2015).

Stakeholder. Stakeholder refers to groups and individuals who has the capacity to influence the failure and success of organizational practices. A stakeholder can include a public employee, managers, the public, and the government (Freeman & Phillips, 2002).

Summary

Corrupt business and management practices within the PHS of Cameroon is of increasing concern among the public and policy makers causing extra financial burden, reduced life expectancy, prevalence of HIV/AIDS and cholera among young adults and inequalities in the geographic distribution of healthcare personnel in rural areas (Kankeu et al., 2016; Osifo, 2014; Yamb & Bayemi, 2017). Such practices within the PHS occurs in several forms and at all levels within the system such as the theft and sale of anti-retroviral drugs used in treating patients with HIV/AIDS which are supposed to be free, demands for bribe payments as a condition for receiving better treatment at in-patient facilities and bribes payments paid by employees to managers to maintain a "nice" position (Kankeu et al., 2016; Osifo, 2014; Yamb & Bayemi, 2017).

Because of the corrupt business and management practices that continue to lead to increased monetary cost to individuals, delays in seeking preventative care within the PHS and suggestions for additional investigations into such practices (Kankeu et al., 2016; Osifo, 2014; Njong & Ngantcha, 2013; Tinyami et al., 2016; Yamb & Bayemi, 2017) uncovering the perceptions of key stakeholders in diminishing the problem was needed (Harrison et al., 2015; Kankeu et al., 2016; Yamb & Bayemi, 2017). To accomplish the purpose of the study and provide an answer to the problem the occurrence of corrupt practices at all levels within the PHS, stakeholder theory guided the study by explaining the perceptions of key stakeholders (nurse managers, nurses and physicians) within the context of organizational governance of how to diminish corrupt practices.

Stakeholder theory is an organizational management theory in understanding how the actions of stakeholders, including (nurse mangers, nurses and physicians) impact the success of an organization (Freeman, 1984; Freeman & Phillips, 2002). In understanding the perceptions of stakeholders, this study used the multiple case study design and semi-structured interviews as it facilitated the understanding of contextual meanings within the study setting (Clarke & Braun, 2017; Kvale, 2986; Yin, 2009). By examination the perceptions of stakeholders, it increased our understanding of why such corrupt business and management practices occur and potential solutions in diminishing it (Kankeu et al., 2016; Osifo, 2014; Tinyami et al., 2016; Yamb & Bayemi, 2017).

Chapter 2

Literature Review

The realization that corrupt business and management practices exists at all levels within the PHS of Cameroon and leading to increased monetary cost to individuals and delays in seeking preventative care, spawned the need for a theoretical framework in understanding how individuals or groups within an agency can affect or be affected by the organizational management processes (Freeman, 1984; Kankeu, Boyer, Toukam & Abu-Zaineh, 2016; Yamb & Bayemi, 2016). Stakeholder theory (ST) was used for understanding stakeholders' perceptions of how to diminish corruptive practices (Freeman, 1984).

ST was the preferred framework in investigating and understanding stakeholders' perceptions because it offered a platform in constructing a corpus of scholarly contributions of key stakeholder perceptions from within the various realms, the different forms of corrupt business and management practices and at all levels within the PHS (Freeman, 1984; Harrison et al., 2015; Kankeu et al., 2016; Ngoran & Ngantcha, 2013; Yamb & Bayemi, 2017). Because key stakeholders operate or are qualified to operate within each specific realm and are likely to have the greatest amount of insight as to how to diminish corruption from within their specific realms, an understanding of key stakeholders' perceptions per realm is the best means in diminishing corruptive practices (Freeman, 1984; Harrison et al., 2015). Thus, the understanding of key stakeholder perceptions of all forms of corruption yielded relevant understandings, views and suggestions designed to diminish it (Tormusa & Idom, 2016; Yamb & Bayemi, 2017).

Background of stakeholder theory

ST is a normative management approach for understanding the actions and/or behaviors of individuals and groups within the context of organizational management and was developed and popularized by Edward Freeman (Freeman, 1984; Miles, 2017; Njong & Ngantcha, 2013; Tantalo & Priem, 2014). Though the conceptualization and development of stakeholder theory is largely credited to Freeman (Hasnas, 2013; Tantalo & Priem, 2014; Zhong, Wang & Yang, 2017) scholars (Brown & Foster, 2013; Freeman, 1984; Gonin, 2015; Hühn & Dierksmeier, 2016; Kurz, 2015) have traced the origins of the ideas shaping stakeholder to Adam Smith's arguments about moral actions and self-interest behaviors of business owners and its effects on business relationships, among individuals and the general public.

Smith's (1776) arguments were that because the natural inclination of business owners is to maximize profits by selling their products at a price that yields the most profit per unit cost they may become unaware of the consequences of such actions to its customers and their own survival as customers may choose to not buy again. Smith's supposition was that, it is in the best interest of the business owner to sell his/her products in a way that is economically profitable to both parties by selling at a price that the customer can afford because its helps in building and enhancing business relationships between the parties as the customer may return to buy more (Brown & Foster, 2013; Freeman, 1984; Gonin, 2015; Smith, 1776).

Following Smith (1776) and in the aftermath of the great depression as corporations grew in size, scholarly attention shifted to self-interest behavior of managers in relation to organizational management (Barnard, 1938; Berle & Means, 1932; Freeman, 1984; Harrison, Mishra & Mishra, 2013). The focus of this attention was in the management of the firm and the role of managers and/or directors as the number of shareholders increases with firm size. Specifically, the arguments were that as corporations and its shareholders grew, those who are charged with managing the daily affairs of the firm (managers, directors) may become self-interested by acting in their own advantage if effective means of scrutiny are not put in place (Berle & Means, 1938; Freeman, 1984; Mishra & Mishra, 2013). Because of this, Berle and Means (1932) and Barnard (1938) suggested among others greater accountability and transparency initiatives (reporting, auditing), as well as imbedded voting rights for all shareholders was needed to ensure the actions of managers are aligned with those of the shareholders and to prevent bad management practices. General Electric corporation expanded the shareholder primacy argument of Berle and Means (1932) by defining four main key shareholder groups that are critical to firm success which includes, the general public, shareholders, customers, and employees (Freeman, 1984; Mishra & Mishra, 2013).

Building upon agency management, shareholder synergy and self-interest literature (Brown & Forster, 2013; Tantalo & Priem, 2014) proposed and used a practical legitimacy framework to examine the role of organizations in relation to the public and its stakeholders. In particular, they examined how managers and/or firms can morally prioritize corporate socially responsible (CSR) initiatives while maintaining stakeholder synergy. Brown and Foster (2013) cited the case of Google executives as they contemplated entering the lucrative and untapped internet market in China. The problem faced by Google executives was that censorship is not legal in the U.S. but legal in China and is contrary to the firm's contractual and moral obligations to its user rights policy of free speech as defined in the state of California (U.S.A) where it is incorporated. Using the practical legitimacy (rational consensus with the truth) approach, Brown and Foster (2013) argued that in considering entering the Chinese market Google executives should consider its contractual obligations of providing uncensored information to its home users which is grounded on shared interest as oppose to legitimizing its self-interest of short-term profits.

Within the agency management and shareholder synergy literature, Merton (1957) developed the concept of role set for understanding how an individual's role set (i.e., the responsibilities, actions and behaviors attach to an action in relation to others) may impact the implementation of change processes within an agency (Freeman, 1984; Stuart & Moore, 2017). Stuart and Moore (2017) and Tucker (2014) further expanded on Merton's work by examining power inequalities and interactions of stakeholder relationships within agencies, as well as the role of middle managers in initiating change processes. Using survey data derived from public organizations in the United Kingdom, they revealed that difficulties in enacting changes are a result of conflicts in balancing competing stakeholder interests and identifying proper role sets for each stakeholder such as employees and supervisors (Stuart & Moore, 2017; Tucker, 2014).

Following contributions from role set, change processes and stakeholder relationships, Igor Ansoff (1965) led a team of researchers at the Stanford Research Institute (SRI) in 1963 that worked on a management to help them better understand the nature of team work, agency processes in decision making and problem analysis and its effects on organizational success and performance (Eskerod, Huemann & Savage, 2015; Freeman, 1984; Magill, Quinzii & Rochet, 2015). Ansoff (1965) derived the term *stakeholder* for identifying those groups, including employees, shareholders, customers, suppliers, lenders, and society as the only group whose support is critical for agency success. According to Ansoff (1965) and Freeman & Miles (1984) the term "stakeholder" was used for generalizing the idea

14

of the stockholder as the only group to which management is responsible to (Freeman, 1984; Freeman, Harrison, Wicks, Parmar, & Colle, 2010).

Freeman (1984) drew upon insights from shareholder and stakeholder management literature (Ansoff, 1965; Barnard, 1938; Berle & Means, 1932; Merton, 1957) to reconceptualize stakeholder theory. Freeman (1984) defined a stakeholder as an individual or group, including (customers, suppliers, lenders, policy makers, activist groups, employees and owners) both from within and outside the agency whose support and influence are critical in the success and management of the firm (Freeman, 1984; Hasnas, 2013; Tantalo & Priem, 2014). Freeman's (1984) initial assumption and the key argument of stakeholder theory is that the success of organizations is dependent upon how effective managers can balance the interests of all its stakeholders while developing and maintaining effective relationships in a manner that increases the long-term value of all stakeholders (Harrison et al., 2015; Tantalo & Priem, 2014). Thus, having a profound understanding of stakeholder interests is central in shaping and cultivating better business and management practices (Freeman, 2002; Magill et al., 2015).

The current view of a ST as defined by Freeman (1984) is an encompassing definition that is meant to include all the groups and individuals that can influence or be influenced by a firm's management processes (Brown & Forster, 2013; Freeman, 1984; Harrison et al., 2015; Hasnas, 2013). Freeman's (1984) classified stakeholders in two distinct groups, namely internal groups (employees, suppliers, customers, owners) and external groups (policy makers or governments, activist groups, competitors, lenders, special interest groups, etc.). Freeman's (1984) initial conceptualization of ST, including its definition and classification included 11 stakeholder groups.

15

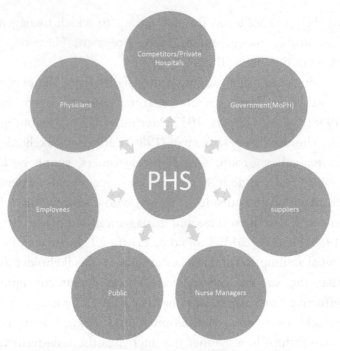

Figure 1. The stakeholder model of the PHS

Since Freeman's (1984) conceptualization of stakeholder theory, scholars (Ferrero et al., 2014; Freeman, 1984; Gonin, 2015; Miles, 2017; Mishra & Mishra, 2013) have provided competing classification, definition and meaning of a stakeholder. For instance, Cleland (1985) defined a stakeholder as an individual with a stake in a project's success. Friend and Hickling (1987) defined a stakeholder as group with a genuine claim on the firm while Wagner (1993) defined a stakeholder as those stakeholders who have a vested interest about decisions made by management. Several authors (Eskerod et al., 2015; Freeman, 1999; Miles, 2017) have argued that such vague definitions hinder the theory's development thus, its applicability in areas such as agency and project management. According to Eskerod et al., (2015) managers may be unable to define and delegate job functions as they may be unable to determine each stakeholder skill set thus, preventing them from effectively collaborating and utilizing their potential to enhance performance (Jo et al., 2016; Mishra & Mishra, 2013; Tantalo & Priem, 2014).

In organizational management, ST is relevant for defining both the key internal and external stakeholders of the hospital system and for informing understanding of each key stakeholders' interests in corrupt practices, motivation or reasoning for other corrupt practices and measures of how to diminish it to enhance success and performance (Freeman, 1984; Tantalo & Priem, 2014; Zhong et al., 2017). Freeman and Phillips (2002) Harrison et al (2015) and Tantalo and Priem (2015) affirmed that stakeholders are relevant to organizations because they are responsible for managing and performing the day-to-day tasks that firms need for providing services to the public and/or customers and thus are at the center in creating value and ensuring long-term success. Freeman (1984) and Hasnas (2013) further argued that the success and performance of an organization is dependent on how well its leaders (managers) can effectively manage the competing interests of all its stakeholders, while building effective relationships. Without such relationships and effective management of competing interests an organization is likely to fail (Freeman, 1984; Harrison et al., 2017; Zhong et al., 2017). Freeman's (1984) definition and classification of ST can be further understood by its three key principles, namely normative, descriptive and instrumental principles (Freeman & Phillips, 2002; Hasnas, 2013; Mishra & Mishra, 2013).

Stakeholder theory. ST is a normative management framework developed and popularized by Freeman (1984) for understanding the actions and responsibilities of individuals and groups within the context of organizational management (Freeman, 1984, Freeman et al., 2013; Hasnas, 2013). Freeman (1984) conceptualized and developed stakeholder theory from a

17

normative perspective that views a stakeholder as a group or individual who can impact or be impacted by the management processes of an agency (Freeman & Phillips, 2012; Miles, 2017) as opposed to the agency or shareholder primacy viewpoint that views a shareholder as key in affecting agency success and to whom management should be responsible.

Freeman's (1984; 1999; 2011) provided an encompassing definition of a stakeholder by describing the relationship and responsibility of an organization to its stakeholders and from the stakeholders to the agency. Freeman (1984) classified stakeholders into two groups: namely main (internal) and general (external) groups. The internal group includes employees, customers, local communities, shareholders, suppliers and distributors and external group, general public, media, activists, business partners, competitors, nongovernmental organizations, policymakers and the government. The main groups are those stakeholders or actors that have a claim to the firm and can directly impact and be impacted by its management processes, while the external groups are those stakeholders that can indirectly impact or be impacted by a firm's management processes and have no direct claim to the firm.

Freeman (1984) contend that the internal groups are vital for the firm's success and advocated management's responsibility in balancing their competing interest while maintaining and building effective relationships for enhancing agency success and survival (Freeman & Phillips, 2002; Harrison et al., 2015). The external groups according to Freeman (1984) are those stakeholders who may indirectly impact or be impacted by the firm's actions and management processes through social activism to demand change. Though Freeman (1984, 2011) provided an encompassing and simple definition of a stakeholder, including its classification the debate surrounding its meaning, definition, and classification continues unabated

(Harrison et al., 2015; Miles, 2017; Mitchell, Agle & Woods, 1997).

On one side, are scholars (Clarkson, 1995; Ferrero, Hoffman, & McNulty, 2014; Friedman & Miles, 2002) that defined, classified and viewed a stakeholder through the primacy lens by classifying stakeholders as shareholders and being the only group to whom management is responsible to and whose interest is critical for firm success (Friedman, & Miles, 2002; Ferrero et al., 2014). On the other side are those (Freeman, 1984; Harrison et al., 2015; Hasnas, 2013) that define, view and classify a stakeholder as any individual or group both from within and outside the firm that can influence agency success either directly or indirectly. Cleland (1985), for example, defined a stakeholder as an individual or group with a vested interest in a project's outcome. Carlon (2014) defines a stakeholder as individuals or groups that have a claim or ownership, rights or interest on the agency and its activities. Friend and Hickling (1987) defined a stakeholder as a group of constituents with a legitimate claim on the firm, while Wagner (1993) defined a stakeholder as an individual or group with a stake about decisions made by the agency. General Electric classified stakeholders as shareholders to include employees, customers and public (Freeman, 1984). Phillips (2003a) distinguishes between derivative (latent and activist stakeholders) and normative stakeholders. Normative stakeholders are those actors to whom the agency has a moral obligation of fairness to (Phillips 2003a). Derivative stakeholders are those stakeholders (competitors, activists) who can either benefit or harm the firm, but to whom the firm has no obligation to (Fassin, 2012; Phillips et al. 2003).

The issue with these viewpoints according to Miles (2017) is that organizations and managers may be unable to determine who are its key stakeholders thus, preventing them from efficiently engage, prioritize and balance stakeholder competing interest while building effective relationships necessary for

19

enhancing performance and success. Heravi, Coffey, and Trigunarsyah (2015) argue that the vagueness in stakeholder definitions and classifications may result in problems with implementing project rules and project processes during its adoption and execution phases, as managers may be unable to properly identify stakeholder responsibilities. Eskerod et al (2015) contend that the vagueness in stakeholder definition may hinder the ability of managers to properly its stakeholder skillsets thus, preventing them from effectively collaborating and utilizing their potential for project realization leading to project delays and cost overruns (Eskerod et al., 2015).

In project management settings and specifically in the manufacturing, healthcare, information technology (IT), and aerospace sectors, that have a higher number of engineering and administrative-related responsibilities, including office secretaries, department managers, and contractors, test engineers, electrical engineers, which are spread across other sub-departments and sub-projects and further managed by multiple stakeholders (managers, employees) proper identification and classification of stakeholders for ensuring efficient task positioning becomes critically relevant for project completion and success (Brady & Davies, 2014; Eskerod et al., 2015; Lucae, Rebentisch, & Oehmen, 2014). A study by Brady and Davies (2014) that investigated how complexities associated with two construction projects (the Heathrow Terminal 5 runway and the London 2012 Olympic Park) was addressed revealed that poor stakeholder identification of contracting and sub-engineering partners were among the reasons why London Olympic Park resulted to cost overruns, delays in opening the Heathrow Terminal 5 runway. Poor stakeholder identification and management also led to flight cancellations and a public relations disaster for British Airways (Brady & Davies, 2014; Tashman & Raelin, 2013). Because of this, Brady and Davies (2014) suggest adopting a collaborative behavioral approach, which identifies stakeholder groups, builds support, creates collaboration, rewards performance and incentives for managing and exposing potential risks. In addition, they contend adopting an integrated workforce approach that includes: clients, engineers, suppliers, and first tier contractors, staff training and development for building a collaborative culture thus, enhancing project success and performance

Lucae et al (2014) affirmed organizations can be negatively impacted without thoroughly identifying their stakeholders because stakeholder responsibilities, needs, interests, and goals may not be properly documented and identified during the initial project planning, adoption and implementation phase thus, leading to project delays. Eskerod et al (2015) argue that proper stakeholder identification is relevant for eliminating potential problems and issues that may occur before, during and after the project thus, minimizing the potential failures and enhancing its success. According to Brady and Davies (2014) Eskerod et al (2015), when stakeholders are not properly identified and engaged in agency processes, the potential for project failure increases. In a related study, Tashman and Raelin (2013) developed the concept of *stakeholder salience to the firm* to account for stakeholders who should matter to the agency and its management, even when agency managers do not perceive them as important and revealed that stakeholders are often not properly identified by managers because of the several meanings and definitions of the term *stakeholder*. However, Tashman and Raelin (2013) did not substantiate in their study what definitions managers used to identify their stakeholders, nor addressed how not having key stakeholders negatively affected project performance and success.

In contrast, Allen, Alleyne, Farmer, McRae, and Turner (2014) investigated the factors frequently critical for assisting with project success and failure using the examples of Proctor & Gamble's New Growth Factory and the U.S. Coast Guard's 123-

21

Foot Patrol Boat project. The findings revealed that stakeholders are often poorly identified because project managers and stakeholders have conflicting stakeholder interests such as opposing opinions over the prioritization of project activities rather than failures in properly identifying stakeholders. According to Allen et al (2014) project managers tend to reject opinions of stakeholders they think will discourage their project plans. The study also revealed that project failures were due to conflicts of interest in career advancement goals between projects managers and stakeholders and not due failures in identifying stakeholders. The studies imply that creating a collaborative culture among stakeholder groups is relevant for not only properly identifying its key stakeholders but enhances the organization's ability to prevent conflicts between its stakeholders as stakeholders see themselves as members rather than rivals (Allen et al., 2014; Brady & Davies, 2014; Tashman & Raelin, 2013). Within the context of PHS management, properly identifying and enhancing synergy between key stakeholders (nurses, nurse managers and physicians') may result in proper task positioning and leading to efficiency in the response rate for answering patient calls for assistance (Hope, 2015; Yamb & Bayemi, 2017). Stakeholder identification and classification has also evolved to include the stakeholder salience model (i.e., the most important stakeholder) in relation to stakeholder proximity and ability to impact agency processes (Mitchell et al., Fassin, 2012).

Stakeholder salience. Mitchell et al (1997) classified stakeholders in terms of their salience in relation to their ability for influencing agency and management processes as primary versus secondary stakeholders. Primary stakeholders are those groups or individuals that can directly impact or be impacted by the agency and having a direct contractual relationship (legitimacy) with the agency, including employees, customers, stockholders, lenders, suppliers, or anyone with a financial interest in the agency (Mitchell et al., 1997; Fassin, 2012). Secondary stakeholders are those groups or individuals, including activist groups, media, regulators and general public with an indirect relationship to the agency but may impact agency activities through protests actions and media scrutiny.

Mitchell et al (1997) developed stakeholder salience model for helping managers identify, analyze and prioritize stakeholder competing needs, interests and priority. Mitchell et al (1997) contend stakeholder salience is relevant for identifying stakeholder competing needs in terms of their salience (i.e., the most important stakeholder) and distinguished three distinct salience models: urgency (stakeholders' ability to initiate or demand immediate attention), legitimacy (the extent to which a stakeholder based on societal norms, including contract and fundamental rights' can claim legitimacy on the agency) and power (the extent to which stakeholders can exert influence on agency and management processes) as the three major stakeholder attributes (p. 864).

According to Mitchell et al (1997), the extent to which stakeholders have all three attributes will determine management's prioritized attention of their claims. The higher the stakeholder salience the higher the priority for attention given to the stakeholder. Researchers (Eskerod et al., 2015; Tashman & Raelin, 2013) affirmed the three attributes compels managers to pay particular attention to stakeholder views and suggestions. Stakeholder salience model is relevant for understanding stakeholder proximity to managers and has been applied in several areas of public management, including project management, healthcare, and information technology settings (Eskerod et al., 2015; Khurram, & Petit, 2017; Magness, 2008; Mattingly, 2014; Tashman & Raelin, 2013) with one attribute having more influence on agency activities than another.

Khurram and Petit (2017) examined the dynamics of stakeholders' salience within the microfinance sector in Pakistan in distinguishable phases of the institutional change process and revealed that power attribute was more important than legitimacy and urgency for encouraging micro finance loan managers to include full and proper disclosure about fees and interest rates on loans. The results also showed that changes in stakeholders' salience are directly related to changes in stakeholders' attributes (power, legitimacy and urgency) suggesting that microfinance stakeholders received the most attention in effecting changes by having the most attributes. The study findings were limited in that it did not delineated the stakeholder groups rather assuming the various groups are homogenous. A similar study by Mattingly (2004) that investigated the relevance of firm-level interactions with sociopolitical stakeholders for explaining agency chances to survive revealed that when firms consider the suggestions of its sociopolitical stakeholders, it positively impacts its social performance, but not its financial performance. The suggestions imply that stakeholder salience maybe relevant for decision making only in some instance, but not all (Mattingly, 2004; Tashman, & Raelin, 2013). Bundy, Shropshire and Bucholtz (2013) suggest stakeholder saliency may also dependent on the type and size of the firm because large organizations compared to small ones have additional complexities in managing several other managers and stakeholders and must effectively prioritize their attention based on the three attributes.

Magness (2008) also used Mitchell et al. (1997) stakeholder salience framework to examine the reactions or responses of two stakeholder groups (management groups) during an environmental disaster. The groups consist of managerial (stakeholder) and investor decision-making (shareholder). Investor-decision response was examined in terms of changing risk and share returns; whereas managerial response was through changes in disclosure (Magness, 2008). The findings revealed that both groups reacted to the disaster at different times, with management responding to the first disaster but not the second while shareholders responded only to the second disaster alone. The results suggest that stakeholder salience though relevant for influencing change may depend on the firm's immediate priority, implying that a firm's survival maybe more important than responding to the needs of its stakeholders when in crisis mode (Eskerod et al., 2015; Magness, 2008). The Stakeholder salience model maybe useful for the current study by informing management in prioritizing attention to their stakeholder suggestions and perceptions of how to prevent and diminish corruption (Stamati et al., 2015; Tashman & Raelin). Tashman & Raelin (2013) suggests management's prioritized attention to stakeholder claims not resulting to success and performance may be due to management's inability to properly interpret the stakeholder's claim. Stakeholder salience is also useful for allowing management to effectively prioritized competing stakeholder claims by proactively placing emphasis on specific attributes thus, facilitating the adoption and implementation of rules, regulations and policies design to enhance agency success and performance (Eskerod et al., 2015; Stamati et al., 2015; Tashman & Raelin, 2013). Freeman's (1984, 1999, 2011) stakeholder theory has also evolved to delineate three distinct principles, including the normative, descriptive and instrumental for understanding management actions and responsibilities within the context of agency management (Donaldson & Preston, 1995; Harrison et al., 2015; Oates, 2013).

Stakeholder normative principle. The normative principle and the core of ST explains management's responsibilities to the agency and its stakeholders and from the stakeholders to the agency for building long-term agency success and value creation (Donaldson & Preston, 1995; Freeman, 1984; Tantalo & Priem, 2014). Freeman (1984, 1999, 2011) developed the stakeholder theory from a normative approach and argues that to enhance agency success and ensure its long-term survival, managers must effectively balance competing stakeholder interests while building effective relationships. Freeman's (1984, 2011) stakeholder normative approach advocates treating all stakeholders fairly. Harrison et al (2015) contend that an agency that manages for its stakeholders ensures its survivability and success.

The normative framework posits that being responsible to stakeholders enhances stakeholder collaboration and increases agency value and performance (Cording, Harrison, Hoskisson & Jonsen, 2014; Freeman, 2007; Tantalo et Priem, 2014). This suggests that how PHS managers (nurse managers) treats its nurses may impact their attitudes and behaviors for providing better care services (Kankeu et al., 2016; Yamb & Bayemi, 2017) and how the hospital system acts towards the communities in which it operates impacts their behaviors and attitudes of the citizens towards the hospital system (Harrison et al., 2015; King, 2015). Stakeholder management responsibilities involves balancing competing interests and giving equal consideration to all stakeholders in terms of policy implementation and decision-making in a way that creates value for all stakeholders and ensures the survival of the agency (Donaldson & Preston, 1995; Freeman, 1984).

In other words, management makes decisions based on stakeholders' fundamental rights (i.e., contract law) and legal rights, and general well-being (Freeman, 1984; Purnell & Freeman, 2012). Since Freeman's (1984) conceptualization of stakeholder theory, there appears a controversy by some scholars (Brown & Foster, 2013; Chan et al., 2014) who have attempted to equate stakeholder theory to corporate social responsibility (CSR). Though Freeman (2011) acknowledges how stakeholder theory might be conceived as CSR because it advocates treating and considering all stakeholders interests in making agency decisions, Freeman (2011) argued stakeholder theory is an agency management theory, not CSR (Freeman et

26

al., 2013; Harrison et al., 2015). This study employed the normative stakeholder approach in understanding the behavior and responsibilities of the PHS and managers towards its stakeholders (Freeman, 1984, 1999, 2011; Donaldson & Preston, 1995; Harrison et al., 2015). The researcher used the stakeholder framework to analyze agency management processes with respect to public management in several settings, including project management, information technology, healthcare and public management (Eskerod et al., 2015; Popescu, 2013; Tashman & Raelin, 2013).

The normative framework explains how the organization and the stakeholders should work together so that they can achieve organizational goals. The agreement between the stakeholders and the firm is based on the firm's ethical principles which govern the relationship between the organization and the stakeholders thus, the normative principle lies in between the descriptive and instrumental principles as it examines agency actions and responsibilities between stakeholders (Freeman 2011; Harrison et al., 2015; Tantalo & Priem, 2014). The normative principle's core hinges on management's decisions and how it impacts stakeholder interest and agency outcomes. Freeman (2011) and Tantalo and Priem (2014) observed that when management's actions affects another stakeholder, then the agency has a responsibility to ensure its ethics principles guides its actions. King (2015) contend that agency decisions should consider the interest of all stakeholders by engaging and soliciting their opinions. This implies management actions that does not consider the interests, views, perceptions and suggestions of its stakeholder may be unethical (Donaldson & Preston, 1995; Fassin, 2012). Thus, the agency should not ignore the interests of its stakeholders just because they do not align with those of management (Freeman et al., 2013; Harrison et al., 2015). The stakeholder normative framework has developed to become one of the most widely used approaches for understanding the responsibilities and actions of managers within the context of agency and public management and has been applied in several settings such as general management, information technology (IT), business ethics and social responsibility, and stakeholder management (Ayuso et al., 2014; Christensen et al., 2015; Mishra & Mishra, 2013; Starks et al., 2015).

Starks et al., (2015) investigated the impact of stakeholder engagement and input, by soliciting the perceptions of relevant stakeholder groups (steering committee meetings, consultations with tribal health system leaderships and tribal subject review committees) for adopting and implementing a depression screening program in Alaska. The solicited perceptions yielded relevant viewpoints and suggestion that enabled local authorities to develop a software-based iPad-tool for better managing depression by emphasizing the role of local culture and family in managing and improving depression outcomes (Starks et al., 2015). In addition, the extensive stakeholder engagement also facilitated the development of a patient-centric approach for managing depression whereby health providers (doctors, pharmacists, nurses) would discuss treatment options, care management and prevention options with patients during office visits (Starks et al., 2015). However, the study did not specify or distinguish between the stakeholder groups (e.g., primary versus secondary). Because of this, it was not clear if the success of the depression program was achieved through stakeholder involvement alone or through protest action from activist groups (media).

A similar study by King (2015) that examined the role of local groups in demanding social accountability revealed that in agricultural societies characterized by semi-authoritarian regimes, revealed that it is the collection of local activists that is most impactful in shaping social accountability outcomes. In contrast, Heravi, et al (2015) evaluated the extent to which key stakeholders are currently involved with planning processes of residential building projects. The findings revealed that engaging stakeholders in construction project management and planning processes led to delays, cost overruns and failures due to conflicting viewpoints and problems in identifying stakeholder roles. The studies suggest that before including stakeholders in agency processes, management should carefully identify key stakeholder skill sets and perspectives from the beginning, thus increasing the prospects for ensuring program success (Heravi et al., 2015; King, 2015; Starks et al., 2015). The normative stakeholder framework has also been applied in studies in the area of public management (Ayuso et al., 2014; Chan et al., 2014; Christensen et al., 2015).

Ayuso et al (2014) examined the relationship between quality management practices in the form of public financial disclosures and its impact on agency performance. The results showed a significant and positive relationship between a firm's financial disclosure records and increase in level of confidence among stakeholders leading to a high degree of trust among investors. At a general level, the results revealed a positive relationship between level of quality management practices which suggests that organizations with higher activities of quality management practices and complying with financial disclosure requirements are more likely to be more socially responsible to both its internal and external stakeholders than those with poor or very low corporate governance practices. The study results are similar to a study by Chan et al (2014) that investigated the role of financial disclosure and corporate governance quality. The study findings showed that firms that consistently apply good governance as an agency strategy are more likely to enhance their performance and value creation for its stakeholders than those that do not (Brown & Forster, 2013; Chan et al., 2014; Tantalo & Priem, 2014).

While the study results were significant, they were limited in that it cannot be generalized to other settings because it was not comparative as it did not include organizations from other countries for comparing differences between the constructs (Chan et al., 2014). Also, the authors did not specify the quality management practices that may be more useful for smaller firms as opposed to larger firms as small firms are not financially positioned to implement all of the quality governance initiatives because they do not have the financial resources as large firms as Jizi et al., (2014) suggested. Chan et al (2014) further suggested that, rather than mandate specific disclosures, managers, policy makers and regulators should focus on initiating quality management activities as a means for enhancing transparent disclosures. The practical implications for the current research are two folds. First, in terms of building stakeholder synergy and trust, information gleaned about compliance in financial disclosures may be useful for management and policy makers for designing policies and rules that addresses the issue of an independent financial reporting board (Brown & Forster, 2013; Chan et al., 2014; Jizi et al., 2014). Second, as part of management's ethical responsibility they should ensure that financial disclosures statements as reported by managers are reflective of the agency's actual performance as opposed to information designed to help its self-image (Christensen et al., 2014; Jizi et al., 2014).

Though these studies revealed a positive relationship between good governance practices and firm performance, similar studies by Christensen at al., (2015) that investigated the extent to which the implementation of good governance practices as mandated by the Australian Securities Exchange Commission (a securities exchange supervisory and monitoring government agency) improves agency performance between large and small firms. The study revealed no relationship between quality governance in the form of financial transparency and performance. Overall, the results suggest that instituting good governance practices may be affected by an agency's own financial status and size and not by its desire for non-compliance (Steamer, 2014). Because of this, Steamer (2014) suggests that firms with limited financial resources should only comply with those transparency initiatives that are mandated by the government. Applying the stakeholder framework in this study may benefit the theory in several areas such as (a) identifying and implementing policies design to enhance efficiency in delivering better healthcare services at in-patient and outpatient facilities in reference, regional and sub-regional hospitals, (b) implementing regulations and procedures design to enhance transparency in the selection process, including hiring, promoting and transferring and (c) adopting policies and initiatives design to enhance attendance and work rules, including absenteeism and tardiness (Asongu, 2013; Fry, 2016). Additionally, the elicited insights of stakeholders may shed more light of potential risk factors that may occur in engendering corrupt business and management practices within the PHS resulting in the implementation of initiatives in identifying and mitigating such potential risks (Fry, 2016; Tormusa & Idom, 2016). The stakeholder theory also delineates the descriptive and instrumental principles.

Stakeholder descriptive/empirical principle. The descriptive principle describes and explains the specific behaviors and characteristics of the organization or how agency and management should act or behave using empirical evidence (Donaldson & Preston, 1995).

Stakeholder instrumental principle. The instrumental principle explains the consequences of management's actions and behaviors to other stakeholders while reemphasizing management's responsibility to the firm and other stakeholders without stipulating specific stakeholders (Donaldson & Preston, 1995).

Stakeholder Management Strategies for Success

Freeman (1984) prescribed several management approaches for helping managers enhance value creation and performance. Strategic management and business practices, involving appropriate agency structure and description of mission statement (stakeholder communication), commitment, management responsibility, total quality management and transparency, including financial disclosures have been shown to positively impact agency performance in both public and private settings (Beschorner, 2014; Chan et al., 2014; Christensen et al., 2015). When good governance practices consisting a combination of policies, rules, laws on ways to manage an agency such as proper financial disclosures requirements and an independent management board, it led to improved performance of Indian and South Korean firms (Gupta & Sharma, 2014). Babnik et al., (2014) investigated the role of mission statements in building firm identity and enhance performance. The authors revealed a positive association between a firm's mission statement and financial performance through five content dimensions: agency concern for stakeholders, alignment towards stability, alignment towards cooperation, orientation towards advancement success, and customer satisfaction. Babnik et al (2014) suggested that mission statements should incorporate agency values, as well as cultural value dimensions, and should inform both internal and external stakeholders.

Other stakeholder theorists (Freeman, 1984; King et al., 2014) have argued that mission statements should be used as a strategic management tool in aligning agency core values and principles with success, including those of its stakeholders. King et al (2014) defined a mission statement as a formal statement of an agency's values and objectives. According to Babnik et al (2014) a mission statement serves as an important agency and management tool for reporting its "core values" and "reason for being" in keeping with its organizational culture (p. 612). Typically, an agency's mission statement describes who is involved (customers, lenders and suppliers), what the agency produces and/or sell (services or products), where it is served (market, public), why it is offered (philosophy/values), how it is offered (distinguishing factors/content dimensions) and how the public should construe the organization's identity or image being projected (Pearce & David, 1987).

King et al (2014) suggest using a mission statement as a preferred agency management tool for communicating agency values; however, the contention includes specific descriptions for better alignment with corporate identity and practices. Harrison et al (2015) have cautioned against over-attention to stakeholders through mission statements to the detriment of the agency and management primary responsibility of creating stakeholder value and balancing interests that could undermine its survival. Babnik et al (2014) and Freeman (1984) suggest the necessity to specify the agency's stakeholders' needs by addressing it in the language of the mission statement. However, such suggestions have resulted to more debate as other researchers (Donaldson & Preston, 1995; Freeman, 1984; King, 2015; Miles, 2017; Mitchell et al., 1997) don't always agree on a specific definition of who or what is a stakeholder (internal versus external) or which stakeholder group should be included. Mitchell et al (1997) for instance, argue that external stakeholders with legitimate claims on the agency should only be determined according to their salience on the agency relative to its relevance to society. King et al., (2014) and Freeman (1984) affirmed management's responsibility in balancing such competing differences in planning and adopting a mission statement relevant to the agency's goals. Freeman (1984) and Norman (2015) also affirmed the Rawlsian strategy for stakeholder management.

33

Freeman (1984) suggest the Rawlsian strategy developed by John Rawls (1971) in his book *The Theory of Justice* as an agency management approach for managers to view themselves as agents of change. Rawls' (1971) initial arguments were focused on inequalities in the distribution of justice, as well as goods and services and its impact on individual liberties and social attainment (Norman, 2015). Rawls (1971) argued that such societal inequalities can be justified if it raises the status of the most vulnerable groups or individuals to ensure they achieve equal or improved social status (Freeman, 1984; Norman, 2015). Within the context of this paper, an interpretation and application of Rawls' (1971) theory would dictate that management of the PHS would view themselves as change agents by ensuring its management and business practices relating to employment (selection and hiring) promotions, transfers, absenteeism and delivery of care services are transparent and are accordance with its own core principles and values to ensure equal opportunity to all of its stakeholders, specifically its least well-off stakeholders (citizens of Cameroon; Freeman, 1984; Norman, 2015).

According to Freeman (1984) and Norman (2015) to effectively implement the Rawlsian approach, managers should begin by sharing the underlying values of the theory by demonstrating their commitment to the principles of justice and equality towards all stakeholders irrespective of their salience (Mitchell et al., 1997). Norman (2015) further suggests management should begin by acknowledging agency inefficiencies that currently exist and be courageous in the ability of management in addressing it. Other Rawlsian theorists Singer (2015) have argued against the applicability of Rawlsian theory in agency management because organizations cannot be considered primarily as a solution for agency problems or conflicts among stakeholders and between stakeholders (external versus internal). In keeping with the Rawlsian debate,

Welch and Ly (2017) affirmed the use of Rawlsian strategy in agency management because the agency occupies key part of public's productive system of social cooperation. According to Welch and Ly (2017), Rawls' suggestions of social equality in a free market society is characterized by private property ownership and democracy, raises critical issues of legitimate agency owners in terms of separation and control. Another management strategy that has been suggested and has been widely used is the concept of stakeholder engagement.

Noland and Phillips (2010) defined stakeholder engagement as management practices that seek to involve stakeholders in a "positive manner" in all aspects involving organizational actions. According to Pandi-Perumal et al., (2015) stakeholder engagement is a two-way process between management and stakeholders that begins when management interacts by communicating with stakeholders to seek information on enhancing agency practices resulting in informed decision-making regarding the adoption, implementation and follow-up of change processes to enhance success. Pandi-Perumal et al., (2015) affirmed the process of engaging stakeholders should be well planned to ensure the intent of the process is to genuinely seek dialog and solutions by ensuring decisions are not made before starting the engagement. In keeping with this affirmation, Noland and Phillips (2010) argued that such guidelines for participation are necessary and important to ensure the intent is not to deceive, rather to receive information from and consult with management on issues affecting stakeholders.

Eskerod et al., (2015) identified five approaches for positively engaging stakeholders namely employee work councils, newsletters, customer focus groups, active public affairs officers and community town meetings. Noland and Phillips (2010) classified stakeholder approaches based on its purpose, manner and method of engagement. Freeman et al., (2007) and Pandi-Perumal (2015) prescribed stakeholder employee work councils and customer focus group as a strategic communication medium for enabling management and stakeholders (both internal and external to interact and seek ideas and solutions about management actions affecting them. Employee work councils and customer focus groups are necessary and important to explain and clarify each stakeholder's role and responsibilities, as well as establishing processes for creating value and success. In addition, customer focus groups are useful for providing stakeholders a setting for expressing their concerns about management practices that directly impacts them and requiring action for addressing it (Pandi-Perumal, 2015).

Using a longitudinal, qualitative, single case method conducted between 2012 and 2015, Eskerod et al (2015) investigated the relationship between stakeholder engagement approaches of a Danish municipal political project in administration, project execution and success. The findings revealed that engagement activities (focus groups and community town hall meetings) are more likely to make stakeholders buy into new council initiatives of tax increase and renovation of public schools; however, the results were mixed when too many stakeholders were included or involved as local managers tend to lose focus of stakeholders. Because of this, Pandi-Perumal et al., (2015) suggest identifying stakeholders' interests, expectations and requirements initially to ensure success. Within the context of agency management, Freeman (1984) and Pandi-Perumal et al., (2015) agree such identification is relevant because stakeholder management encompasses the processes of identifying and classifying stakeholders (internal and external); evaluating stakeholders' skills, knowledge and expertise, as well as determining stakeholder requirements, interests and expectations, communication needs, issues and concerns while maintaining a positive relationship and constantly communicating and interacting with stakeholders about management actions. This study used the stakeholder framework for understanding the perceptions of key stakeholder's interest in corruption, justification of corruption and measures for diminishing it within the public hospital system of Cameroon.

The Public Hospital System (PHS) of Cameroon

Background of the PHS and corruption literature

The PHS is a public institution consisting of several entities, including the national teaching and university hospital known by its French acronym as CUSS, reference hospitals, regional, divisional, and sub-divisional or rural hospitals and pharmacies and managed by the Ministry of Public Health (MoPH; Molem-Christopher et al., 2017; Tinyami et al., 2015). Although the policy framework for establishing a PHS has been traced to a presidential degree No89/011 in 1989 (Molem-Christopher, et al., 2017) the events shaping its establishment has been shaped by a number of factors (Baker, 2015; Fongwa, 2002; Nana, 2016; Nguemegne, 2011).

Fongwa (2002) cited the poor state of the nation's healthcare and a lack of a systematized healthcare infrastructure, including health centers, in-patient hospitals and pharmacies following the country's independence in 1961 and 1962 respectively following a long period of colonial rule. According to Fongwa (2002), about 80% of the population in rural areas lacked any form of regularly systematized healthcare. A study by Tinyami et al (2015) that examined shortages and inequalities in the geographic distribution of healthcare personnel in Cameroon revealed that significant inequalities exist in the geographic distribution of qualified and trained health personnel especially in rural areas. It also showed that within the entire nation only one school exist for training physicians and 40 for training other healthcare personnel, with urban areas such as Yaoundé (capital) having the highest with 10 centers, while the North and South regions having only one center.

According to Tinyami et al., (2015), 70 % of the regions in Cameroon had a density of healthcare personnel-to-population of less than 1.5 to a 1,000, suggesting an acute shortage of healthcare workers. The shortage of healthcare personnel especially in rural areas has been attributed to poor living and working conditions, and fewer prospects for career advancement leading to the documented migration of physicians and nurses to other urban areas and abroad (Tinyami et al., 2015; Yamb & Bayemi, 2017). Shortages and inequalities in the geographic distribution of healthcare personnel and regularly systematized care has been cited as a factor in the high rate of mortality rate of neonates of 95 per 1,000 live birth and infants under five years in the country, as well as the prevalence of malaria in rural areas (Tinyami et al., 2015, p. 6).

Baker (2015) cited the poor state of the country's education following its colonial epoch as a factor that has contributed to shortages in qualified healthcare personnel. Baker (2015) and Fongwa (2002) contend inefficiencies in staff training is due to the lack of an effective educational system for training health personnel resulting to inefficiencies in administering healthcare service such as infant immunization programs (Tinyami et al., 2015). According to Fongwa (2002), training for healthcare personnel in Cameroon while similar to those in other parts of the world lacked the depth required to provide the quality of services expected by the public.

As a result of acute shortages of healthcare and qualified staff, most individuals walked long distances to receive medical care only to be met by corrupt, unqualified and inefficiently trained staff, and bad-mannered employees. Researchers (Fongwa, 2002; Kubbe & McBride, 2015; Yamb & Bayemi, 2017) have attributed worker impoliteness, corruption and inefficient training to several factors. Yamb and Bayemi (2017), for example, investigated corruption forms and healthcare provisions within public hospitals in the Douala and Littoral region and revealed that worker corruption may be due to the low pay levels of public employees. Other scholars (Baker, 2015; Fongwa, 2002) suggests worker impoliteness may be due to improper staff training and inadequate task positioning. According to Fongwa (2002) improper staff training and inefficient task positioning are a result of poor management because most licensed nurses in Cameroon while similar to registered nurses (RNs) in the U.S. are trained at the diploma level, thus, lacking the conceptual knowledge necessary to provide the level of services expected by the public compared to their U.S. counterparts.

Nana (2016) examined the education perspectives and its legacy in Africa, and specifically Cameroon and revealed that the training and education of most Cameroonians are fashioned after the French education system, which does not emphasize the wearing of uniforms, respect in administrative rank and cordiality in providing care services (Fongwa, 2002). The study suggests that corruption, improper task positioning and worker impoliteness may be due to its foundational legacy of education. From a stakeholder and management perspective, understandings from these perspectives may inform hospital managers and policy makers to develop new training programs and policies that seek to enhance the skills and competencies of all its staff members thus, preventing and diminishing the likelihood of worker impoliteness and corrupt attitudes (Hope, 2014; Yamb & Bayemi, 2017).

Following the assessment on the state of its healthcare, the government created a national policy framework that established a national health and hospital system and delineating its organizational and management structures under the Ministry of Public Health with four core principles including (a) participation of other socioeconomic development sectors in health, (b) public involvement, (c) full support of local hospital facilities by regional and reference centers, and (d) equal distribution of health resources with a guiding mission to prevent, improve and delivering better health care services to the public (Fongwa, 2002, p. 326; Kankeu et al., 2016; Yamb & Bayemi, 2017). The mission of the PHS was to improve healthcare access, prevent diseases and enhance the quality of services. To realized its core principles and achieve its mission, the PHS was organized in a bureaucratic management model, with top, middle and periphery administrative levels.

The Organization Structures of the PHS and Corruption Forms

Administrative levels. The PHS is organized as a bureaucratic (top, middle and bottom or periphery) model with the MoPH at the top with six executives supporting the ministry (Njong & Ngantcha, 2013; Molem-Christopher et al., 2017). It consists of several entities, organizations and institutions, including a reference hospital or university teaching hospital, 11 regional hospitals, as well as divisional, and sub-divisional or rural hospitals (in-patient and out-patient) facilities and pharmacies (Molem-Christopher et al., 2017; Ongolo-Zogo et al., 2014; Tinyami et al., 2015). Its primary mission and objective are to prevent diseases, improve healthcare outcomes and deliver better healthcare services to the public (Kankeu & Ventelou, 2016; Molem-Christopher et al., 207; Tinyami et al., 2016). To achieve its core mission and objectives, the PHS was organized in three distinct administrative or management levels with delegated tasks that include: (a) top management, (b) middle management (c) periphery or bottom management.

Top management. The top management is responsible for the elaboration of healthcare concepts, strategies, policies, coordination and regulation in the area of health and well-being and supported by six directorates. It involves designing,

40

implementing and managing a coherent health policy for the country for preventing diseases, improving healthcare outcomes and delivering better healthcare services to the public (Kankeu & Ventelou, 2016; Tinyami et al., 2015; Yamb & Bayemi, 2017). In addition, it is responsible for developing and managing the services that are offered to the public at all public healthcare facilities, including, promotions, task delegations, training and development of personnel, immunization programs, procedures, regulations and policies (Molem- Christopher et al., 2017; Ongolo-Zogo et al., 2014). The MoPH is also responsible for the overall management of the various inter-agencies within the hospital system and the National Center for drug acquisition and distribution also referred to as (CENAME; Molem-Christopher et al., 2017; Njong & Ngantcha, 2013; Yamb & Bayemi, 2017).

To achieve its responsibilities the ministry is supported by six directorates and 10 regional health delegates in all ten regions (Fongwa, 2002). Regional delegates are responsible for controlling, supervising, and coordinating health services at each regional level (Fongwa, 2002; Molem-Christopher et al., 2017). Its structures of care include, hospitals in reference and all hospitals (divisional, sub-divisional and community health centers) and pharmacies within each region. Within the top management level healthcare services are managed and provided at six levels, including: (1) community services (outreach programs through healthcare coordinators), (2) hospital facilities (preventive and healing services managed by registered nurse (RNs) or nurse aides and physicians) and (3) sub-divisional hospitals (receive referrals from rural hospitals and other healthcare centers in the sub-division). Most citizens receive healthcare services from Levels 1 through 3; as well as (4) divisional hospitals (managed by the divisional health officers who oversee the healthcare activities of the entire division), (5) regional hospitals (receive referrals from the regions, divisions and sub-divisions), and (6) the regional health delegate (manages the overall healthcare activities) (Fongwa, 2002).

Within the top management tasked with regulating, delegating, and coordinating health policies and programs, including regional, divisional, reference or teaching hospitals, corruption exists in the form of bribes or "informal" payments paid to officials and employees (Kankeu et al., 2016; Njong & Ngantcha, 2013; Osifo, 2014). Family members and patients make these payments themselves as a condition for accessing and receiving better treatment and care services at in-patient facilities, as well as out-patient facilities at reference and teaching hospital (Kankeu et al., 2016, p. 42; Yamb & Bayemi, 2017). In addition, corruption occurs in the theft and sale of drugs like anti-retroviral that has been donated or purchased by the government which are supposed to be free to patients seeking treatments for the Human Immune Virus and Acquired Immune Deficiency Syndrome (HIV/AIDS; Kankeu et al., 2017; Stearns et sl., 2017; Yamb & Bayemi, 2017).

Because of this, it has resulted in extra monetary cost to individuals, as well as their families and delays in seeking medical treatment (Jakubowski et al., 2017; Yamb & Bayemi, 2017). Delays in seeking medical treatment has led to an increase in the number of people especially young adults that are living with HIV/AIDS and early death of children under the age of five dying of preventable illness like malaria (Kankeu & Ventelou, 2016; Hajizadeh et sl., 2014; Tinyami et al., 2015). The middle management or administrative level of the PHS is another area where corruption is occurring.

Middle management. The middle management, is charged with providing technical support in the form of financial allocation and personnel to health districts through regional delegations of public health and having responsibilities to structures like regional hospitals and its equivalents (Molem-Christopher et al., 2017). Within the administration of the PHS, consisting of secretary generals, directors and regional delegates who are responsible for appointing and delegating responsibilities to personnel corruption exists in bribes paid by medical doctors and staff members to superiors to avoid transfers to rural areas and maintaining "nice" positions (Yamb & Bayemi, 2017, p. 98). Such practices which have resulted to an uneven distribution of qualified healthcare personnel especially in rural areas, in the ratio of 1.3 to 1,000 has led to a high rate of neonatal deaths of 95 per 1,000 live births (Montoya et al., 2014; Tinyami et al., 2015). Furthermore, corrupt business practices occur in the abuse of delegated authority by officials in appointing and promoting family and clan members in senior positions without consideration for other prospective applicants irrespective of agency policies against such practices. In addition, corruption occurs in the demands of "informal" monetary payments paid by students and their parents as a condition for admission into the sole medical training college (Okafor et al., 2014; Yamb & Bayemi, 2017).

Such practices deny other qualified potential applicants equal opportunities and results in inefficiencies in the coordination of HIV/AIDS programs and lack of preventive strategies in combatting infectious diseases like cholera and malaria. Because of this, it has led to recent increases in the prevalence of these diseases among children and young adults (Djouma, et al., 2016; Okafor et al., 2014; Yamb & Bayemi, 2017). The periphery management is another level within the PHS where corruption is occurring.

Periphery or bottom management level. The periphery management is tasked with implementing health programs (immunization, wellness) in the country and having responsibilities to structures like health centers, district and sub-divisional hospitals (Molem-Christopher et al., 2017). It consists of frontline employees responsible for day-to-day operations such as infant immunization, maternal outreach and preventive illness programs at district and sub-regional hospitals, as well as community centers. Within the periphery management, corruption exists in unjustified and unexplained tardiness and absence of employees and some officials during normal business hours, while working a second job as managers or directors remain silent (Molem-Christopher et al., 2017; Ongolo-Zogo et al., 2014; Yamb & Bayemi, 2017).

Because of this, it has affected the ability of the PHS to efficiently manage its core mission of improving and delivering better healthcare services to the public and leading to longer wait times in queues to see a doctor, delays in responding to patient calls or requests and increase in nurse and physician workload due to personnel shortage (Kankeu et al., 2016; Kankeu & Ventelou, 2016; Njong & Ngantcha, 2013; Yamb & Bayemi, 2017). Scholars (Gong & Wang, 2013; Luiz & Steward, 2014; Pena-Lopez, 2014; Yazan, 2015) have identified several contextual factors (culture, history, education) and political factors (judicial, political system) for understanding the public's perceptions of corruption and initiatives for diminishing it. For years researchers (Hechanova et al., 2014; Hofstede & Hofstede, 2005; Pena-López & Sánchez-Santos, 2014; Quah, 2014) have used several contextual factors, including a country's culture, political system, legal system, gender in understanding the public's perceptions of corruption and initiatives for diminishing it and relevant to this study.

Contextual Factors and Corruption Perspectives

Legal system. Contextual factors such as the type and structure of a country's legal system may affect individual perceptions and assessment of corruption thus, affecting anti-corruption initiatives design to diminish it (Hope, 2014; Kim, 2014; Pellegrini & Gerlagh, 2017). Kim (2014), for example, examined anti-corruption initiatives in 200 countries and its effects on corruption using the legal-administrative approach, which focuses among others on a country's enforcement of the rule of law, instituting administrative reforms, regulations, separation of governmental affairs from politics, anti-favoritism, and protection for whistle-blowers to encourage citizens to report incidence of corruption thus, reducing corruption in public institutions. The findings revealed that legal-administrative approaches are significant in preventing and reducing corruption. The results also showed that countries in North America (United States, Canada) and Europe have less corruption than those in developing nations.

Kim (2014) contented that countries in North America and Europe have legal systems, that are anchored in strong common law practices that adopt and strictly enforces laws and regulations thus, preventing and diminishing corruption. In addition, Countries in Europe and North America have legal processes, including courts, police that require officials to efficiently execute corruption laws using both internal and external control measures, including, accounting, auditing, and program evaluation, whereas in developing countries such legal-administrative approaches are non-existent as politicians are able to influence the legal and administrative processes design to prevent corruption through bribes to gain personal advantage. A similar study by Hope (2014) that investigated the public perceptions of persistent corruption within public hospitals in Kenya and anti-corruption initiatives revealed that the existence of corruption within public hospitals is due to the lack of effectiveness by the country's legal and administrative institutions, including courts, prosecutors, judges, police officers and other public officials to adopt and strictly enforce anti-corruption laws such as whistle blower protection design to encourage public officials and individuals to report incidences of corruption (Hope, 2014).

In contrast, Pellegrini and Gerlagh (2017) revealed no relationship between a country's legal system and corruption. In particular, Pellegrini & Gerlagh (2017) used cross-country data from several developing countries with a history of poor governance practices to investigate the link between corruption and its legal system and revealed that political instability, authoritarian regime, poor governance, and lack of independent press were associated to high levels of corruption, but an insignificant relationship between corruption and a country's legal system. The study suggests that government efficiency is useful in order for anti-corruption initiatives to succeed by strengthening public bureaucracies with competent public officials or agents thus, preventing and mitigating corrupt practices in public agencies (Kim, 2014; Pellegrini, & Gerlagh, 2008; Treisman, 2007). The study also indicates that individuals are less likely to engage in corruption activities when anti-corruption law, policies, regulations such as whistle-blower protection and administrative reforms are anchored in sound legal principles and are strictly enforced both by public officials and employees (Angeles & Neanidis, 2014; Kim, 2014). From a stakeholder perspective, it suggests that when stakeholders perceive agency policies and regulations relating to anti-corruption (whistle-blower protection) are strictly enforced the likelihood of reporting corrupt practices will likely increase, as well as their involvement in corruption, thus preventing and diminishing it (Hope, 2014). Additionally, such understandings may inform policy makers and PHS managers to adopt and implement new laws that strengthens enforcement and punishment for corrupt behavior. Culture a contextual factor that has been used for understanding public perceptions, views and understandings about corruption and anti-corruption initiatives relevant to this study.

Culture. The use of culture as a concept in this study is because of its encompassing nature in shaping societal and individual attitudes, actions, behaviors, perceptions about corruption and efforts to diminish it. Authors (Pena-López & Sánchez-Santos, 2014; Yaza, 2015) affirmed that knowledge can be a product of social construction especially with individuals and their attachment with believes, norms and practices. According to Hofstede and Hofstede (2005), the definition and approach to mitigating corruption are dependent on culture because of its capacity for influencing the norms of society. How individuals perceive cultural norms and its influence on corruption has been applied in studies in both public and private management settings (Hechanova et al., 2016; Lewellyn & Bao, 2017).

Hechanova et al (2014) investigated the linkages between culture building dimensions and its relationship to workplace culture of corruption within public hospitals in Philippine and revealed that management communication of agency values and norms were significantly positive in shaping employee attitudes and behavior towards corruption. This is because, employees get their cues from agency officials about what is right or wrong. They suggested that managers should constantly communicate agency values of customer satisfaction and corruption mitigation to employees and lead by example to prevent and diminish the corruption (Hechanova et al., 2014; Lewellyn & Bao, 2017).

This study is in keeping with that of Lewellyn and Bao (2017) that examined the role of national culture and corruption. In particular, they investigated the role of culture in managing financial earnings and statements around the world and revealed that when agency officials continuously reinforce agency values of best practices relating to proper financial disclosures, it strengthens employee attitudes about ensuring such financial results are reflective of the agency's financial performance, thus building stakeholder confidence about such results thus, ensuring stakeholder value creation and agency performance (Lewellyn & Bao, Luiz & Steward, 2014). However, the findings are contrary to a similar study by Owoye and Bissessar (2014) that examined the continued occurrence of corruption in Sub-Sahara Africa (SSA) through the lens of leadership style and its influence on governance and institutional failures. They revealed that persistent corruption in SSA is a result of dictatorial regimes that limit press freedom, thus preventing its citizens from actively engage in the fight against corruption rather than its national culture.

The use of culture as a construct in understanding citizens' perceptions about corruption and corruption mitigation efforts has also been studied with often conflicting results (Donchev & Ujhelyi, 2014; Pena-López & Sánchez-Santos, 2014; Udechukwu & Mujtaba, 2013). Donchev and Ujhelyi (2014) examined the extent to which factors such as individual perceptions and country sociocultural characteristics (culture, religion, political system) may affect levels of corruption specifically in cross-country studies. They revealed that individual perception and experience of corruption is a weak predictor of reported corruption (Donchev & Ujhelyi, 2014). It also showed that some of the factors often used as indicators of low occurrence of corruption, including economic development and good governance, methodically bias corruption perception indices downward from corruption experience (Donchev & Ujhelyi, 2014, p. 328). This is because, corruption indices are often misleading due to their failures in properly measuring corruption activities. Donchev and Ujhelyi (2014) further argue that what constitutes corruption varies from one country to another as corrupt practices are often shrouded in secrecy and are hard to observe and measure (Donchev & Ujhelyi, 2014). In contrast, Udechukwu and Mujtaba (2013) contended that although giving a small gift to a public official for performing a service is a custom or norm in countries like Cameroon and Nigeria it may be considered as a corrupt or illegal act in the United States. Overall, the findings suggest that using corruption perception indices as a measure of corruption indicator and experience may be more problematic than suggested as corrupt experiences are country specific.

From a stakeholder perspective, culture creates an understanding and perception to public organizations and individuals due to its encompassing capacity for influencing the norms, values and beliefs of individuals (Freeman, 1984; Hofstede & Hofstede, 2005). Thus, culture might be useful for understanding the divergent perceptions, views and insights of key stakeholders about their experiences of corrupt business and management practices and suggestions of how to diminish it. In addition, the resultant understandings from stakeholder's views, suggestions and experiences about corruption and measures to mitigate it might be useful for PHS managers and policy makers to adopt new policies and regulations design to prevent and diminish corruption (Njong & Ngantcha, 2013; Osifo, 2014). Demographic characteristics such as education and gender are contextual factors that have been used for understanding the stakeholder perceptions about corruption and anti-corruption initiatives.

Education. Researchers have considered education as a factor for influencing individual perceptions about corruption and assessment of policies to diminish it (Fortunato & Panizza, 2015; Walton & Peiffer, 2017). Authors (Fortunato & Panizza, 2015; Walton & Peiffer, 2017) examined levels of education among individuals as an independent construct for understanding public perceptions and evaluation of corruption and anti-corruption measures in public and private institutions. Walton and Peiffer (2017), for example, showed that levels of education positively influenced public assessment of corrupt practices in public institutions. In particular, they revealed that educated individuals (with at least a college education, college diploma) are more likely to report corrupt activities to authorities than less educated ones.

A similar study by Fortunato and Panizza (2015) that investigated the relationship between education and corruption revealed a significant relationship between levels of education and good governance practices. The studies imply that improving the education level of employees and citizens may be a strategy that policy makers and agency management might consider for preventing and diminishing corrupt practices. From a PHS management viewpoint, the findings suggest that adopting and implementing training programs that seek to develop the human development capacities of stakeholders (employees) might be useful to enable employee and stakeholder awareness about corruption and its impact on agency success and value creation (Fortunato & Panizza, 2015; Walton & Peiffer, 2017). When stakeholders (nurses, nurse managers, physicians) are educated and informed they are more likely to monitor and report corrupt practices to appropriate management and government officials thus, diminishing its likelihood of occurring (Fortunato & Panizza, 2015; Walton & Peiffer, 2017). In addition, education, enable individuals to have an awareness and interest in ensuring best business practices, including merit based selection, hiring and promotion policies are strictly enforced thus, leading to less corruption (Chidi, 2014). Chidi (2014) suggests that individuals with higher levels of educations might have the potential to perceive corruption and assess ways to diminish it better than those with lower education levels. Gender perspectives is another factor that has also been examined for influencing individual perceptions about corruption and efforts to diminish it.

Gender. Gender perspectives in understanding corruption and initiatives in diminishing it has come under scrutiny in the scholarship (Ionescu, 2014; Iroghama, 2011). Ionescu (2014) used gender as a construct for investigating its role in the failure of anti-corruption initiatives in multinational institutions and revealed that anti-corruption efforts that considered the opinions and suggestions of women were more likely to succeed because women instill a sense of integrity in workplace settings, thus are more likely to provide suggestions for preventing and diminishing corruption. The result indicates that including gender perspectives on the anti-corruption efforts resulted in a more balanced approach to enforcing anti-corruption efforts. In keeping with this suggestion, a similar study by Iroghama (2011) that examined the public perceptions of government success in fighting corruption in Nigeria, revealed that the women are more responsive in assessing anti-corruption initiatives better than men. In contrast, a similar study by Merwe and Harris (2012) that examined the perceptions of university students on public sector corruption revealed that men are more likely than women in assessing and rating anti-corruption initiatives than women. The findings were limited in that it did not explain the primary gender attitudes that may have influenced participant responses. Thus, further qualitative studies that take into account gender perspectives should consider gender attitudes in participant responses. Overall, the studies suggest that gender perspectives can be useful for understanding stakeholder perceptions about corruption business and management practices within the PHS and efforts to diminish it. Political characteristics (governance) have been used for understanding its influence on societal and individual perceptions of corruption and mitigation efforts.

Political factors and corruption perspectives

Political system. The quality of governance in the form of independent or free media, independent legal institutions (courts, police) and type of government (single party, or multi-party) are relevant for understanding individual perceptions about corruption and anti-corruption initiatives (Agbiboa, 2012; Quah, 2015; Yamb & Bayemi, 2017). Quah (2015) investigated the link between corruption and quality of governance by comparing the corruption experiences of six Asian countries (Brunei Darussalam, Cambodia, Myanmar, Pakistan, Papua New Guinea (PNG) and Vietnam) to explain their levels of success in mitigating corruption by dividing the quality of governance and type of government into three categories namely (high, medium, and low) level of quality governance. The findings revealed a positive relationship between the type and quality of governance in the form of (free media, independent courts, multi-party democracy) and level of corruption in public institutions especially in Brunei.

The results also revealed that countries with a low or small quality of governance practices are more likely to have high levels of corruption as seen in countries such as Vietnam and Pakistan. Nations with a medium level of quality governance had a manageable or moderate level of corruption, while those with a good or high degree of quality governance showed a weak degree of public corruption like in Brunei. The study implies that quality governance might be a reason in the high levels of corruption within public institutions in most developing countries. To substantiate this argument, Quah (2015) cited the United States as an example that have a well-structured governance structure, with checks and balances amongst its branches of government (executive, judiciary, legislative) that have a low degree of corruption (public) because the structure serves as a measure of checks and balances for preventing corruption.

This study is similar to that by Kubbe and McBride (2015) that analyzed the propensity by individuals to engage in and to punish corrupt behavior in a three-person sequential move-game and revealed that countries with a high degree of press freedom, democratic political systems and independent judicial system (courts, police) tend to have successes with anti-corruption policies than those with single-party political systems or autocratic system of governance. According to Kubbe and

McBride (2015), democratic institutions protects and ensures the likelihood of motivating citizens to actively participate in anti-corruption initiatives without fear of reprisal thus, reducing its possibility of occurring. From a stakeholder perspective, it implies that individuals living in countries with good quality governance and democratic political systems might be more willing to express their perceptions and views freely about corrupt activities and to report corrupt activities compared to those in authoritarian countries thus, affecting anti-corruption efforts.

In contrast, the link between good governance (political system) and levels of corruption has been a contentious issue. In examining the factors associated with citizens' perceptions of a country's economic conditions, Safadi and Lombe (2013) argued that a country's quality of governance cannot be used as a measure for shaping citizens views about corruption because authoritarian states have a capacity to achieve a low-level of public corruption by instituting strict controls on corruption thus, preventing its likelihood of occurring. Though the results were significant, the study only investigated public corruption mitigation from the institutional perspective that only examines corruption mitigation supported by political leaders with strict laws and emphasis on imprisonment of corrupt officials while having limited focus on corruption activities and mitigation efforts by non-public officials.

Researchers (Safadi & Lombe, 2013; Quah, 2015) suggests that the success of anti-corruption initiatives in countries with poor governance quality may be more dependent on the commitment of its citizens rather than its leaders and public institutions such as legislature. Studies (Luiz & Steward, 2014; Nguemegne, 2011; Osifo, 2014) that have assessed the effectiveness of anti-corruption initiatives in SSA, including Cameroon and Nigeria have revealed corruption as prevalent because political leaders lack the political will to enforce anti-corruption laws and initiatives and for slowing down anti-corruption initiatives by arresting political opponents rather than corrupt officials with close personal connections.

Summary

The understanding that corrupt business and management practices exists at all levels within the PHS and leading to increased monetary cost to individuals and delays in seeking preventative care, spawned the need for a theoretical framework in understanding how individuals or groups within an agency can affect or be affected by the firm's management processes (Freeman, 1984; Kankeu et sl., 2016; Yamb & Bayemi, 2016). Stakeholder framework undergirded this study by providing a compendium studies for understanding stakeholders' actions and responsibilities to the firm and other stakeholders (Freeman, 1984). ST was the preferred framework for investigating and understanding the perceptions of stakeholders' because it offers a platform in constructing a corpus of scholarly contributions of key stakeholder perceptions from diverse realms within the PHS (Freeman, 1984; Harrison et al., 2015; Kankeu et al., 2016; Ngoran & Ngantcha, 2013; Yamb & Bayemi, 2017).

Because key stakeholders (nurse managers, nurses and physicians operate or are duly trained and qualified to work within each specific realm and are likely to have the greatest amount of insight of how to prevent and diminish corruption from within their specific realms, an understanding of key stakeholders' perceptions per realm is the best way to diminish corruptive practices (Freeman, 1984; Harrison et al., 2015). The elicited understanding of key stakeholder views, suggestions and perceptions of all forms of corruption yielded relevant suggestions and ways to diminish corruption (Tormusa & Idom, 2016; Yamb & Bayemi, 2017).

Stakeholder theory is a normative management approach that was conceptualized, developed and popularized by Freeman (1984) for understanding the responsibilities and actions of individuals and groups (stakeholders) within the context of agency management (Freeman, 1984; Miles, 2017; Njong & Ngantcha, 2013; Tantalo & Priem, 2014). While Freeman (1984) has been largely credited with the theory's development and conceptualization, the ideas shaping it has been traced to Adam Smith's (1776) foundational work in the *Wealth of Nations*. Smiths' (1776) arguments were that because the natural inclination of business owners is to maximize profits by selling their products at a price that yields the most profit per unit cost they may become unaware of the consequences of such actions to its customers and their own survival as customers may choose to not buy again.

In the aftermath of the Great Depression, as corporations grew in size the need to protect the shareholders' interest became important as the number of shareholders also increased. Because of this Berle and Means (1932) suggested greater accountability and transparency initiatives for protecting shareholders. Following contributions from Berle and Means (1932) a management team at Stanford Research Institute (SRI) working under Igor Ansoff coined the term "*stakeholder*" for helping them better understand the nature of team work, agency processes in decision making and problem analysis and its effects on organizational success and performance. Freeman (1984) drew upon the work of Igor Ansoff to reconceptualize the term *stakeholder* into stakeholder theory (Hasnas, 2013; Tantalo & Priem, 2014).

Freeman (1984) defined a stakeholder as an individual or group, including (customers, suppliers, lenders, policy makers, activist groups, employees and owners) both from within and outside the agency whose support and influence are critical in the success and management of the firm. Since its conceptualization researchers (Donaldson & Preston, 1995) provided competing definitions of a stakeholder based on the contextual setting of their studies. For example, Cleland (1985) defined a stakeholder as an individual with a vested interest in a project's outcome. Friend and Hickling (1987) defined a stakeholder as group of constituents with a legitimate claim on the agency while Wagner (1993) defined a stakeholder as those group or individuals who have a stake about decisions made by the organization.

The issue with these definitions according to Miles (2017) is that organizations and managers may be unable to determine who are its key stakeholders thus, hindering their ability to engage, prioritize and balance stakeholder competing interest for building effective relationships necessary to enhance its performance and success. In project management settings and specifically in the manufacturing, healthcare, information technology (IT) and aerospace sectors, that have a higher number of engineering and administrative-related responsibilities, including office secretaries, department managers, and contractors, test engineers, electrical engineers, which are spread across other sub-departments and sub-projects and further managed by multiple stakeholders (managers, employees) proper identification, classification of stakeholders for ensuring efficient task positioning becomes critically relevant for project completion and success (Eskerod et al., 2015; Heravi et al., 2015; Lucae et al., 2014). Stakeholder identification and classification has also evolved to include the stakeholder salience model (i.e., the most important stakeholder (Mitchell et al., 1997; Fassin, 2012).

Mitchell et al (1997) developed stakeholder salience model for helping managers identify, analyze and prioritize stakeholder competing needs, interests and priority. Mitchell et al (1997) contend stakeholder salience is relevant for identifying stakeholder competing needs in terms of their salience (i.e., the most important stakeholder) and distinguished three distinct salience models: urgency (stakeholders' ability to initiate or demand immediate attention), legitimacy (the extent to which a stakeholder based on societal norms, including contract and fundamental rights' can claim legitimacy on the agency) and power (the extent to which stakeholders can exert influence on agency and management processes) as the three major stakeholder attributes (p. 864). According to Mitchell et al (1997) the extent to which stakeholders have all three attributes will determine management's prioritized attention of their claims. The higher the stakeholder salience the higher the priority for attention given to the stakeholder. stakeholder theory has also evolved to delineate three distinct principles, including the normative, descriptive and instrumental principles for understanding management actions and responsibilities within the context of agency management (Donaldson & Preston, 1995; Harrison et al., 2015; Oates, 2013).

The normative principle and the core of stakeholder theory explains management's responsibilities to the agency and its stakeholders and from the stakeholders to the agency for building long-term agency success and value creation (Donaldson & Preston, 1995; Freeman, 1984; Tantalo & Priem, 2014). Freeman (1984, 1999, 2011) developed the stakeholder theory from a normative approach and argues that in order to enhance agency success and ensure its long-term success, managers must effectively balance competing stakeholder interests while building effective relationships. Freeman's (1984, 2011) stakeholder normative approach advocates treating all stakeholders fairly. Harrison et al (2015) contend that an agency that manages for its stakeholders ensures its survivability and success. The Normative framework explains how the organization and the stakeholders should work together so that they can achieve organizational goals. The agreement between the stakeholders and the firm is based on the firm's ethical

57

principles which governs the relationship between the organization and the stakeholders thus, the normative principle lies in between the descriptive and instrumental principles as it examines agency actions and responsibilities between stakeholders. The stakeholder normative principle has been widely used by scholars in several studies in public management settings, including project management and public administration. This study used the stakeholder principle to investigate the perceptions of key stakeholders' interest in corruption, justification for corruption and measures of how to diminish it.

The PHS is a public institution consisting of several entities, including the national teaching and university hospital known by its French acronym as CUSS, reference hospitals, regional, divisional, and sub-divisional or rural hospitals and pharmacies and managed by the Ministry of Public Health (MoPH; Molem-Christopher et sl., 2017; Tinyami et al., 2015). The policy framework for establishing a PHS has been traced to a presidential degree No89/011 in 1989 (Molem-Christopher, et al., 2017). The factors preceding its creation has been traced to several factors.

Fongwa (2002) cited the poor state of the nation's healthcare and a lack of a systematized healthcare infrastructure, including health centers, in-patient hospitals and pharmacies. According to Fongwa (2002) about 80% of the population in rural areas lacked any form of regularly systematized healthcare. According to Tinyami et al (2015), 70 % of the regions had a density of health personnel-to-population of less than 1.5 to a 1,000, suggesting an acute shortage of healthcare workers. The shortage of healthcare personnel especially in rural areas has been attributed to living and working conditions, and few prospects for career advancement leading to the documented migration of physicians and nurses to other urban areas and abroad. Baker (2015) cited the poor state of the country's education following its colonial epoch as a factor that has contributed to unqualified, inefficiently trained and shortages in healthcare staff. Baker (2015) and Fongwa (2002) contend inefficiencies in staff training is due to the lack of an effective educational system for training health personnel resulting to poor management and affecting the quality of care services provided if it exists. According to Fongwa (2002) training for healthcare personnel in Cameroon while similar to those in other parts of the world lacked the depth required to provide the quality of services expected by the public.

To access healthcare services, most individuals walked long distances only to be met by corrupt, unqualified, inefficiently trained staff, and bad-mannered employees. Researchers (Fongwa, 2002; Kubbe & McBride, 2015; Yamb & Bayemi, 2017) have attributed worker impoliteness, corruption and inefficient training to several factors. Following an assessment on the state of its healthcare, the government created a national policy framework that established a national health and hospital system and delineating its organizational and management structures under the Ministry of Public Health. The mission of the PHS was to improve healthcare access, prevent diseases and enhance the quality of services. To realized its core principles and achieve its mission, the PHS was organized in a bureaucratic management model, with top, middle and periphery administrative levels.

The top management, is responsible for the elaboration of healthcare concepts, strategies, policies, coordination and regulation in the area of health and well-being and supported by six directorates. With the top management, for example, corruption exists in the form of bribes or "informal" payments paid to officials and employees (Kankeu et al., 2016; Njong & Ngantcha, 2013; Osifo, 2014). Family members and patients make these payments themselves as a condition for accessing and receiving better treatment and care services at in-patient facilities, as well as out-patient facilities at reference and teaching hospital. Because of this, it has resulted in extra monetary cost to individuals, as well as their families and delays in seeking medical treatment (Jakubowski et al., 2017; Yamb & Bayemi, 2017). Delays in seeking medical treatment has led to an increase in the number of people especially young adults that are living with HIV/AIDS and early death of children under the age of five dying of preventable illness like malaria. For years studies (Hechanova et al., 2014; Hofstede & Hofstede, 2005; Quah, 2014) have used contextual factors, including a country's culture, political system, legal system, gender in understanding the public's perceptions of corruption and initiatives for diminishing it and relevant to this study.

Culture is a concept that has been used for understanding its influence on individual and societal perceptions of corruption. Culture is used as an encompassing factor in shaping societal and individual attitudes, actions, behaviors, perceptions about corruption and efforts to diminish it. Authors (Pena-López & Sánchez-Santos, 2014; Yaza, 2015) affirmed that knowledge can be a product of social construction especially with individuals and their attachment with believes, norms, and practices. According to Hofstede and Hofstede (2005), the definition and approach to mitigating corruption is dependent on culture because of its capacity for influencing the norms of society. How individuals perceive cultural norms and its influence on corruption has been applied in studies in both public and private management settings.

Chapter 3

Research Method

Research Methodology and Design

A qualitative, multiple case study research method with semi-structured interviews were selected in investigating key stakeholders' (nurse managers, nurses and physicians) perceptions of how to diminish corrupt business and management practices in the PHS of Cameroon. A qualitative, multiple case study design was selected for its facilitative capacity in providing understandings of each stakeholders' perception in diminishing corrupt business and management practices, something which would be hard to achieve using an experiment in a controlled setting (Yin, 2009). Also, case study allowed for interviewing key stakeholders in a naturalistic environment, private offices of nurse managers, physicians and homes of nurses or where appropriate. Thus, yielding relevant insights into stakeholders' perceptions (Yin, 2009). Additionally, case study was selected because it allowed for the inclusion of several data sources such as interviews, written notes, and observations in providing robustness (Houghton et al., 2013).

Yin (2009) defined a case study as an in-depth study of a particular phenomenon within their contextual setting. A case study may involve one or more units including a single person (a case) or a group of people (multiple cases; Yin, 2009). This study used the multiple case method involving three of each (nurse managers, nurses and physicians) in understanding their perceptions of corrupt business and management practices within their specific realms in the PHS of Cameroon. The multi-case method was selected because it allowed the researcher in solicitating direct responses of participant perceptions about corrupt business and management practices in their contextual setting, something which would have been hard to achieve using a quantitative experimental method involving numerical data (Yin, 2009). Also, the multiple case design assisted the researcher in receiving robust information about participant interest in corruptive practices and associated problems in diminishing it thus, enabling policies and regulations designed to mitigate it. The case study method further allowed the researcher to collect data from multiple sources, including semi-structured interviews and transcriptions, as well as written notes (Yin, 2013a). Kvale (1983) and (Yin, 2009) suggested that semi-structured interviews and notes are appropriate methods in collecting qualitative case study data.

Despite the positive arguments against qualitative data as being unscientific because of its subjectivity and use of non-numerically quantifiable data, Kvale (1996) argued that qualitative interviews are neither subjective nor objective because they are conducted in interpersonal settings where objectivity itself can be subjective. Though semi-structured, interviews were used in soliciting direct responses from participants to open-ended interview questions, written notes of each interview session, including details of participants (location, date, time and position title) were also taken before, during and after the interview sessions where appropriate for detail analysis (Kvale, 1983; Yin, 2013a). Case study analysis may involve one or more units (Yin, 2009). In this study, each individual participant constituted a unit of analysis for a total of nine cases. As such, the analysis included each individual unit and multi-unit as a whole. For the analysis, the qualitative, deductive thematic analysis method was used.

The qualitative, deductive thematic analysis was used because of its facilitative capacity in discovering patterns of themes within the data set, something which would be hard to achieve using a thematic discourse analysis as it describes patterns across the entire qualitative data (Clarke & Braun, 2017). The thematic analysis involved transcribing each participant recorded responses verbatim into a Microsoft Word document and notes in generating initial codes, including searching for themes, reviewing and defining similar themes within the data set to describe participant perceptions of the phenomena in relation to the research questions (Clarke & Braun, 2006; 2017). The thematic analysis included each unit and multi-units as a whole. The units allowed for the thematic analysis of each individual unit and multi units as a whole, as well as thematic analysis of the relationships between the units. The thematic analysis of the diverse set of participants three of each (nurse managers, nurses and physicians) yielded relevant understandings, views and insights in answering the research questions and thus, achieving the study's purpose (Stake, 1985; Yin, 2009). Clarke and Braun's (2017) organized phases was used for conducting the thematic analysis.

The six phases of thematic analysis included (1) a recursive review and familiarization with the data and taking side notes, (2) using open and axial coding in establishing categories, (3) identifying categories into themes and sub-themes, (4) reviewing and refining similar themes, (5) defining and naming themes and (6) describing and reporting participant perceptions of the phenomena in relation to the research questions (Clarke & Braun, 2006; Yin, 2009).

The data set comprised of all the individual interviews and responses to each interview question and written notes (Clarke & Braun, 2006; Yin, 2009). The primary role of the researcher was to recursively review and code the data line by line and using open and axial coding method thus, enabling the selected extracts to be classified, tagged, and matched with the organized extracts (Clarke & Braun, 2006; Yin, 2009). The researcher applied axial coding, the matching of themes to sub-themes for analysis (Clarke & Braun, 2017). The researcher was active in identifying the codes as the codes are progressively abstracted at higher levels, the process of originating and categorizing codes in facilitating the identification of themes (Clarke & Braun, 2006; 2017; Yin, 2009). Where similarities in participant responses are noted, supporting quotations are extracted.

During coding, content validity, the cross-checking of participant responses to interview questions was used in ensuring credibility and reliability of the study (Kvale, 1996; Yin, 2009). According to Kvale (1996), content validity is achieved when the core of a response to an interview question is similar among three or more participants. Thus, the higher the number of matching responses, the higher the content validity (Kvale, 1996). The data analysis process, included coding, selecting, naming, labeling, and extracting to produce an axial framework thus, encompassing a detail description of the data set and subtle accounts of the response themes (Clarke & Braun, 2006, pp. 87-93; Yin, 2009). Thus, the case study method and particularly, the semi-structured interviews facilitated the achievement of the study's goal of how to diminish corrupt business and management practices within the PHS. While Braun and Clarke's comprehensive set was used in analyzing and coding the data, Yin's (2009) organized protocol was used for the study's design because it provided a detailed and comprehensive process in conducting the study.

The steps to the study design included (a) refining the interview questions through field testing based at least three hospital directors (Kvale, 2008), (b) recruitment of participants using the convenience and purposive sampling process, (c) conducting the case study semi-structured open-ended interviews, including recorded transcription of participant responses and written notes and (d) using theoretical deductive thematic analysis in interpreting and answering the research questions (Clarke & Braun, 2017; Yin, 2009). The first step to the design involved selecting at least three expert reviewers (hospital directors) and using the purposive sampling process to conduct field testing of the research questions. It involved locating and calling directors of regional hospitals in the Northwest region of Cameroon until at least three separate hospital directors agreed to work as expert reviewers and establishing contacts. A formal package containing a letter of introduction, interview questions and description about the constructs used in developing the term *perception* (insights, views, understandings) in ensuring proper descriptor of the term was emailed to each reviewer.

Purposive sampling was used to select participants and involved searching, locating and contacting (emailing and calling) stakeholders listed in the hospital personnel directory until nine potential participants agreed to be interviewed. Potential participants were mailed or emailed a formal letter of introduction, including intent to participate, informed consent form and instructions and scheduled interview dates-initiated schedules (Yin, 2009).

Third, the case study semi-structured interviews were initiated in the private offices of participants or personal settings where appropriate and using a digital Samsung Galaxy Note 4 in recording participant responses, including written notes. Kvale's (1986) interview protocol suggests the importance of using an interview script in opening and closing interviews and a note or face pad in recording details of the interview, including date, time, location, and participant title or position. Each individual interview was recorded using a Samsung Galaxy Note 4 digital audio recorder (Kvale, 1996). Semi-structured interviews were conducted in the private offices and non-agency settings and based on the participant's discretion, and through telephone sessions.

Fourth, each participant responses were transcribed verbatim, including written notes for analysis and using the deductive thematic analysis (Clarke, 2017). Thematic deductive analysis was selected because of its facilitative capacity in the discovery of themes (Clarke & Braun, 2017; Yin, 2009). The analysis involved transcribing each participant recorded responses and notes in generating initial codes, including searching for themes, reviewing and defining similar themes within the data set to describe participant perceptions of the phenomena in relation to the research questions (Clarke & Braun, 2017).

Throughout the coding and analysis phases, the researcher took steps to avoid the potential for researcher bias by ensuring that the report of the findings was accurate and reflected the responses of participants. This was done by postponing the identification of the hidden aspects of the contents until all the tables were completed, thus mitigating the chances for bias by the researcher. Kvale (1996) further suggests several forms of triangulation in qualitative case studies. Data triangulation occurs when participant responses are consistent with others in the data set such as written notes. The researcher compared the contents of the written notes to look for fluidity in answering the questions as suggestive of straightforwardness and confidence.

Population

The target population included males and females ranging from 21-60 years, the legal age in Cameroon (Mbuagbaw et al., 2011). The population was employees working at the largest public hospital, situated in the Northwest region of Cameroon. The hospital population consisted of all the employees within the hospital. The estimated population size of nurse managers relevant to the study consisted of a total of 10 participants (N=10). The estimated population size of nurses relevant to the study consisted a total of 40 (N=40). The estimated population size of physicians relevant to the study consisted of 20 (N=20). Using the convenience and purposive sampling process, the researcher selected a total of nine participants from each population each of which would have been employed for at least one year at the hospital at the time of selection. The selected population of each set meeting the study's criteria was nine participants, including three nurse managers (N=3), three nurses (N=3) and three physicians (N=3). The nurse managers who were part of the study are part of the management team and had worked for at least five years within the hospital. Their primary functions included managing and supervising the overall process in ensuring policies, procedures and initiatives are properly implemented to ensure better outcomes in patient well-being. This includes managing and supervising the daily functions of nurses, nurse aides and other care givers within their department to ensure they are administering medications, following immunization guidelines for infants and promoting wellness outcomes (Helfat & Martin, 2015).

Nurse Managers are trained at local vocational or health science college and have at least a higher national diploma, equivalent to a bachelor degree and certified by at least one board (Eta et al., 2011; Helfat & Martin, 2015). The management-level requirement for nurse managers (Yamb & Bayemi, 2017) grew because of the nature of corrupt management practices as such activities are often shady and involved acts that are interlaced with agency policies and complex laws (Johnston, 2014). Thus, studies have selected management level participants with better understandings of corruptive practices for soliciting their perceptions about agency and/or corrupt practices (Harris & Merwe; 2012; Naystand et al., 2013; Yamb & Bayemi, 2017). Nurses are equally trained in local vocational colleges or health science colleges and have an equivalent of an associate's degree or high school diploma and certified by at least a nursing board (Eta et al., 2011; Helfat &

Martin, 2015). Nurses are primarily responsible among others for administering medicines, performing immunizations for infants and ensuring patients are taking their prescribed medicines, as well as for processing patients to see a physician (Eta et al., 2011). Physicians working in the hospital system had undergone and completed an organized training program at an accredited medical college and had a degree in general medicine and/or specialty and certified by at least a medical board (Helfat & Martin, 2015). Physicians work at various agency realms and/or administrative level relevant to their specialty. The physician's role within the hospital system is multi-faceted and includes, assessing patient history to provide the best form of treatment and outcome, providing continuous care to patients, including referrals to other care facilities and specialists to treat and improve patient well-being (Tang et al., 2013).

Sample

The purposive and convenience sampling methods were used in recruiting participants. Kvale (1986) and Yin (2013a) suggested purposive sampling as a suitable method in soliciting direct responses to open-ended interview questions with predefined characteristics and for its appropriateness in yielding the most pertinent and rich data. Within the context of this study, the purposive and convenience sampling method were used in recruiting a distinct and diverse set of key stakeholders who work or are knowledgeable about corrupt business and management practices in a specific real and an administrative level within the PHS (Yin, 2009). The purposive sampling of managers was limited to nurse managers. The purposive sampling of employees was limited to nurses and physicians. The purposive sampling of expert witnesses was limited to hospital directors (Yin, 2013a). Also, only participants who are working at a regional hospital and situated in the region of Northwest of Cameroon were included in the sample.

Recruitment for the proposed purposive sample involved searching and locating the names, position title and contact information (email and cell phone) and using the directory listing of hospital personnel as Internet search listings such as yellow pages are nonexistent in Cameroon (Darley, 2003). The researcher avoided recruiting participants with whom there exist a relationship and with whom the researcher had a personal knowledge. For a multiple case study, Yin (2009) affirmed a range of six to 10 interviews, with six being the lowest number of interviews required in achieving saturation. If the recruited sample did not meet the requirement for saturation recruitment would have continued until saturation requirement was satisfied (Yin, 2009). Yin's (2013a) argument for the suggested minimum number of interviews is because of the need for sufficiently rich data and for satisfying saturation requirement. For this study, a total of nine participants were interviewed, including interviews with three nurse managers, three nurses and three physicians. Aside from purposive sampling, the convenience sampling method was used in the recruitment process as well.

The convenience sampling method involved contacting (calling and emailing) potential stakeholders (nurse managers, nurses and physicians) located in the personnel directory of the regional hospital until the required sample size was achieved so that nine participants agreed to be interviewed. Yin's (2009) argument for a minimum of six to 10 interviews is because of the need for yielding sufficiently rich data. According to Kvale (2008) and Yin (2009) the more diverse the content of the interview questions, the greater the number of interviews needed in achieving sufficiently rich data (Kvale, 2008; Yin, 2013a). Upon locating the required number participants three of each (nurse managers, nurses and physicians) for conducting interviews, the researcher-initiated contacts by email and by telephone. Inclusion criteria was limited to participants who consented to participate and provided a reliable contact information for further communication were included (Yin, 2009). Exclusion criteria for the sample included participants who were unable to provide a signed consent form and a reliable information for communication (Yin, 2009).

Materials/Instrumentation

The researcher used semi-structured open-ended questions to gather information needed for the study. The researcher developed a total of nine open-ended interview question, including three sub-questions for the purpose of soliciting responses of stakeholders' perceptions about corrupt business and management practices and measures for diminishing it. The development of the interview questions was guided based on the problem of the study and for yielding sufficiently rich data for answering the research questions (Kvale, 2008; Yin, 2009). The interview questions were developed using Kvale's (2008) seven phases for developing and organizing interview questions.

Based on the first phase, the researcher used several constructs such as interests, motives, rationale, views and insights as appropriate descriptors of the term *perception* for the purpose of soliciting and eliciting key stakeholders' perceptions, views, insights, suggestions and understanding about corrupt business and management practices within the PHS and how to diminish it. Kvale (2008) suggests using open-ended terms for developing the interview questions such as *what* and *how* because it allows participants to provide open-ended responses to the interview questions. Because of this, all of the questions were developed and patterned using the term *how*.

In the second stage of designing and developing the interview questions the researcher ensured that all the questions yielded the expected purpose of the study, which is eliciting sufficient understandings, views, and insights about corruptive practices within the hospital system (Kvale, 2008). As such, the interview questions reflected the research questions of the proposed study. Prior to interviewing, an initial set of interview questions were taking directly from the research questions for field testing based at least three expert reviewers (hospital directors). The expert reviewers (hospital directors) were physicians who work in the hospital and have undergone and completed a training program in a medical college with a degree in medicine and certified by at least a medical board. Hospital directors manage the overall functions of the hospital system by ensuring policies, procedures, initiatives and regulations design to eliminate corruptive practices and improve agencies services, including proving optimal patient care services, selecting and hiring qualified staffs and eliminating "informal" or bribe payments in seeking better services are effectively implemented across the various agency realms and administrative units (Yamb & Bayemi, 2017).

The criteria for selecting the expert reviewers were based on their level of experience from working as a hospital director or other expert level role in a specific agency realm and administrative level within a hospital system. The second criterion for selection was their level of education, preferably with a focus in health sciences. Upon locating (hospital directory) and calling hospital directors until at least three expert reviewers agreed to serve as expert reviewers (an information package containing an introduction letter, stating the purpose of the study, asking consent to participant, the original research questions and the constructs used in developing the term *perception* (interests, views, rationale, justification) was sent to the reviewers. The researcher seek confirmation from the expert reviewers to ascertain if the constructs used for developing the interview questions and for further refining them (interest, motives, rationale, and problems) were appropriate descriptors of the term perception.

Reviewers were asked to indicate their responses using a 5-point Likert Scale ranging from 1 to 5, with 1 being very inappropriate and 5 being very appropriate. Thus, responses scoring 3 and above indicates appropriateness (Pontes & Griffiths, 2015). Aside from feedbacks derived from the rating scale, the researcher elicited specific feedbacks and suggestions from the reviewers. In particular, the researcher asked what changes or modifications can be made to the questions in terms of phrasing, language used, description of terms in order to help make the questions simple and easy to understand. The researcher also asked the reviewers if the questions need to be reordered (so that question one may become question three). Additionally, the researcher asked the reviewers whether there may be a need for adding or reducing the number of questions so as to reduce the length of the interview sessions. Furthermore, the researcher asked the reviewers for ideas and suggestions for follow up and probing questions for the purpose of yielding sufficiently rich data (Kvale, 2008; Yin, 2013a).

The researcher utilized the expertise of the reviewers to further develop the final interview questions to ensure credibility and dependability of the research questions (Kvale, 2008, Yin, 2013a). Yin (2009) suggests that the interview questions should be sufficient in number in yielding rich data relevant in answering the research questions. Using the third or interviewing phase an interview guide was developed for maintaining proper interview procedures and for ensuring each participant is answering the same set of questions thus, ensuring standardization of the entire interview process (Kvale, 2008). Also, the interview guide was structured in a pattern for allowing comfortability and flexibility between participants and the researcher thus, enabling the researcher to ask probing and follow-up questions where possible as sufficient data is optimal and needed for the analysis and for reporting the findings (Kvale, 2008). Furthermore, feedback responses from the expert reviewers and dissertation committee members were incorporated for ensuring credibility and dependability (Kvale, 2008). During the interview process, a face-sheet and an opening and closing script was used for guiding the researcher (Kvale, 1996).

Research Procedures

The procedures for conducting the research involved collecting data using semi-structured interviews with nine stakeholder participants (three nurse managers, three nurses and three physicians). Prior to interviewing, an initial set of interview questions were derived directly from the research questions for field testing based at least three expert reviewers (hospital directors) situated in the Northwest region. The expert reviewers were recruited using purposive and convenience sampling process and involved searching and locating potential the hospital personnel directory and calling until at least three hospital directors agreed to operate as expert reviewers. Feedbacks from expert reviewers were incorporated into the research question in enhancing validity. Each interview (nine total interviews) was independently conducted in the private offices of participants and private non-agency locations where appropriate.

Each interview was recorded using a Samsung Galaxy Note 4 digital recorder having a playback feature, and transcribed verbatim after each session. Prior to recording, the researcher informed and secured participants' consent before recording and placing the recording device on the table. Immediately after each interview, a brief portion was played back to participants in ensuring their vocal intonation. The researcher used a face-sheet and an opening and closing script in guiding the researcher

(Kvale, 1996). The face-sheet was used in recording the circumstances of each interview, including name, time, the participant position title and location (Kvale, 1996). Kvale (1996) suggests that each interview should be transcribed verbatim and confidentially. The researcher also used an interview guide for conducting the interviews (Kvale, 2008).

Data Collection, Processing and Analysis

Semi-structured open-ended interviews were used to collect data from a sample of nine participants, including three nurse managers, three nurses and three physicians. A total of nine interviews were conducted individually in face-to-face sessions, thus allowing the researcher to take written notes of details of the interview such as firmness of handshake and eye contact as an indication of truthfulness. Interview sessions were conducted in the private offices of participants or private non-agency locations where appropriate. For a multiple case study, Yin (2013a) suggests a range of 6-10 interviews, with six being the lowest number of interviews needed to achieve saturation. Each interview session lasted no more than 45 minutes. Each interview was recorded and using a Samsung Galaxy Note 4 digital recorder with playback feature. Kvale (2008) suggests transcribing each interview verbatim after each interview.

Prior to commencing each interview, the researcher informed participants to secure their consent before recording their responses by placing a recording device on the table. Immediately after each interview, a brief portion was played back to participants in ensuring their vocal intonation. During the interview process, a face-sheet and an opening and closing script was used in guiding the researcher (Kvale, 1996). The face-sheet was used in recording the circumstances of each interview, including name, time, position title and location (Kvale, 1996). After each interview the researcher transcribed each audio

74

recording verbatim and saved in a Microsoft Word document in a password protected personal laptop. The researcher notified participants (via informed consent form) that the transcribed files and recordings would be destroyed after seven years, per NCU policy. In addition, the researcher also excluded the names of participants to protect their identities and using pseudo or fake names.

Flexibility was used during the interview process to ensure participants are comfortable thus, enabling follow-up questions. The overarching goal of the open-ended interview questions were to gather sufficient details about the key stakeholders' perceptions, views, assessment, and understandings of corrupt business and management practices within the PHS. The first part of the interview involved an introduction from the researcher. The second part asked participants about their perceptions of the different forms of corrupt business and management practices within the PHS. The goal was to gain much understanding about participant's perceptions and insights regarding corruptive practices within the hospital system. The third part focused on gathering participant's perceptions about other corrupt business and management practices within the PHS. The fourth part was aimed at gathering ways, suggestions and solutions in diminishing such practices. The solicited responses were transcribed for coding and analysis.

For the coding and data analysis the qualitative, deductive thematic analysis was used because of its facilitative capacity in discovering themes or patterns of meaning within the data set, something that would be hard to achieve using a "thematic decomposition analysis that describes patterns across the qualitative data" (Clarke & Braun, 2017). The thematic deductive analysis involved transcribing each participant recorded responses and notes taking in generating initial codes, including searching for themes, reviewing and defining similar themes within the data set to describe participant perceptions of the phenomena in relation to the research questions (Clarke & Braun, 2017). Essentially, Clarke and Braun's (2017) and Yin's (2009) steps and/or procedures for analyzing case study units and sub-units initiated the thematic analysis of each individual unit (individual stakeholder participant) each stakeholder domain (nurse managers, nurses, or physicians), and each sub-unit (including three stakeholders from each domain), and the sample as a whole, as well as the thematic analysis of the relationships between the units with sub-units.

Clarke and Braun (2017) and Yin (2009) organized steps and/or phases for using thematic analysis allowed the researcher to have a dynamic role in understanding the perceptions of participants (stakeholders) in their contextual setting. The six phases of the thematic analysis process included: (1) a recursive review and familiarization with the data and taking side notes, (2) using open and axial coding in establishing categories, (3) identifying categories into themes and sub-themes, (4) reviewing and refining similar themes, (5) defining and naming the themes and (6) describing and reporting participant perceptions of the phenomena in relation to the research questions (Clarke & Braun, 2017; Yin, 2009).

The data set consisted of all the individual data items within the data set (written notes, Microsoft Word document and interview transcriptions); though, individual interviews with responses to each interview question were analyzed as individual data sets (Clarke & Braun, 2017; Yin, 2009). During the coding process, the primary role of the researcher involved a recursive familiarization of the data and coding the data line by line and using open coding (Clarke & Braun, 2017). In the first or initial phase, the researcher recursively reviewed the transcribed responses to become acquainted with the data and categorized the data into codes. The codes were collated into per stakeholder per question in identifying the number and/or percentage of responses to each question. In the second phase, the researcher applied axial coding in establishing potentially matching codes or for analysis and using table development function in Microsoft Excel, as well as axial codes per stakeholder domain per interview question. The axial coding per stakeholder and per stakeholder domain were collated using the table function in Excel as shown in the Findings section of chapter 4 of this study. The arrangement of axial codes enabled the researcher in making comparisons to help identify valid contents such as comparisons of axial codes from amongst the responses of the three different nurse managers to the interview questions, comparisons of axial codes from amongst the responses of the three nurses to the interview questions and comparisons of axial codes from amongst the responses of the three physicians to the interview questions. The researcher expected the comparisons to be suitable in-line with Yin's (2009) process for analyzing units. Kvale (1986) suggests ensuring content validity (the cross-verification of participant responses to interview questions) during the coding and reporting phases. According to Kvale (1986) content validity occurs when the responses among three or more participants are basically the same. Thus, the higher the number of matching responses, the higher the content validity (Kvale, 1996). The researcher verified content validity throughout the axial coding process by ensuring researcher and participant honesty, as well as accuracy in reporting the findings by postponing the identification of the hidden aspects of the contents until all the tables are completed, thus mitigating the chances for bias by the researcher. Kvale (1996) further suggests several forms of triangulation in qualitative case studies. Data triangulation occurs when participant responses are consistent with others in the data set such as written notes. The researcher compared the contents of the written notes to look for a firm handshake and eye contact as suggestive of straightforwardness and confidence. Also, the researcher had designed the interview questions to reflect the research questions.

The researcher expected the coding and extracting to result in an axial framework (an overall idea of the data patterns and its relationships) for identifying the categories into themes and sub-themes (Kvale, 1986; Yin, 2009). In the third phase, the researcher began analyzing the collated codes by combining them to form and overarching theme, as well as sub-theme and using a visual presentation document such as Microsoft Excel for representing the data. The researcher identified the relationships between the codes to identify the main themes and sub-themes between them (Clarke & Braun, 2017). The researcher anticipated finding sets of codes that may not fit well with the main themes and created a new "miscellaneous" theme for such codes (Clarke & Braun, 2017). In the fourth phase, the researcher began reviewing and refining similar themes, including sub themes while looking for data to support them. Because of this, themes without sufficient data to support them were combined to form a single theme while others were separated into several other themes. According to Clarke and Braun (2017) internal and external data homogeneity (the meaningful cohesion between themes) should be clear in order to properly identify themes.

Because of this, the researcher conducted two levels of reviews and refinement of the themes by reading all the organized extracts for each theme to ensure they form a coherent pattern (Clarke & Braun, 2017). If the main themes form a consistent pattern, the refinement of themes commenced; however, if the main themes are not in a consistent pattern, the researcher checked to see if there are problems with the themes or within the data extracts. This involved rearranging the themes to create a new theme. The refinement of the themes and sub-themes were similar to the processes mentioned in this phase; however, it was done in relation to the entire data set and in consideration of the validity of the individual themes (Clarke & Braun, 2017). The refinement of the themes and sub-themes were to ensure they form a coherent pattern that can be easily identified and named.

In the fifth phase of the coding process, the researcher began defining the themes to analyze the data. Essentially, it meant identifying what each theme and sub-theme is about in order to determine the aspects of the data that are captured within them and for naming it (Clarke & Braun, 2017). In this phase, the researcher identified concise names for the themes and sub-themes to easily identify and give readers an idea of what they are (Clarke & Braun, 2017). The researcher accomplished this by recursively going over the collated data extracts for each theme to name and arrange them in a coherent account that form a coherent pattern and using accompanying narrative based on supporting data. For each theme and sub-theme, a detailed narrative was provided to tell a concise and non-repetitive story about them and more importantly, to fit with the overarching story of the research purpose and for describing and reporting the findings (Clarke & Braun, 2017; Yin, 2009).

In phase six, the researcher conducted a final analysis of the finished themes and its sub-themes to ensure it is supported by the data extracts in order to report the findings. The researcher's role was to provide a concise and compelling narrative account of the story based on the data in a way that is non- repetitive, logical and convincing (Clarke & Braun, 2017; Yin, 2009). As such, the findings provided enough evidence and clear examples of the themes within the data extracts to show its occurrence in the themes.

Assumptions

The assumptions were that the selected research method qualitative, multiple case study was best for the study as it allowed the researcher in eliciting and yielding relevant stakeholder perceptions about the corruptive business and management practices in the PHS and measures in diminishing it. The second assumption was that the selected sample is a true representative of the PHS and having working knowledge and lived experiences about corrupt business and management practices within each specific agency. As part of the selection criterion for the study, the researcher recruited key stakeholders by searching and locating participants and using hospital personnel directory. Because the generalization of study findings is dependent on truly representative samples selecting a diverse and distinct set of key stakeholders was relevant.

Limitations

A potential limitation for this study was that of bias as participants may not be truthful and honest with their responses because of sensitivities in discussing a topic like corruption and thus, affecting external validity in generalizing the findings. This limitation was overcome by scheduling one-on-one interviews in the private offices of participants and private locations where appropriate. In addition, per NCU and IRB policies, participants were assured of confidentiality in participating and safeguards in securing the data in a password-protected private laptop and data destruction after seven years. Another limitation was that of researcher bias (Yin, 2009).

Researcher bias in qualitative studies may occur during coding, analysis and reporting phases (Kvale, 2008; Yin, 2009). Because of this, the researcher mitigated bias by taking steps in order to ensure the report of the findings were accurate and reflected the responses of participants. This was done by postponing the identification of the hidden aspects of the contents until all the tables were completed, thus mitigating the chances for bias by the researcher. Kvale (1996) further suggests several forms of triangulation in qualitative case studies. Data triangulation occurs when participant responses are consistent with others in the data set such as written notes. As such, the researcher compared the contents of the written notes with the recorded responses to look for straightforwardness and confidence in answering the interview questions.

Delimitations

Delimitations included the geographic setting of the study, the qualitative, multiple case study method and the convenience, the selected participants and purposive sampling process are the established boundaries of this study (Davis, 2013). The study investigated the perceptions of key stakeholders who work or have knowledge about corrupt business and management practices in the PHS of Cameroon. In particular, the qualitative, multiple case study research design was selected for its facilitative capacity in soliciting the perceptions of key stakeholders about corruptive business and management practices and measures in diminishing it. Using the convenience and purposive sampling process, a sample including key stakeholders (three nurse managers, three nurses and three physicians) who work or have knowledge about corrupt business and management practices within a specific agency were selected.

Summary

A qualitative, multiple case study, including semi-structured interviews was conducted individually in face-to-face sessions for the purpose of investigating corruptive business and management practices within the PHS of Cameroon. The case study method was selected for its facilitative capacity in discovering themes within the data set (Clark & Braun, 2017; Yin, 2009). In particular, this study investigated key stakeholders' perceptions about corrupt business and management practices

81

within the PHS and measures in diminishing it (Kankeu et al., 2016; Tinyami et al., 2016; Yamb & Bayemi, 2017; Yin, 2009). Prior to interviewing an initial set of questions were derived directly from the research questions for field testing based at least three expert hospital directors in ensuring validity of the research questions to the interview questions (Yin, 2009).

The population for this study included a distinct and diverse set of nine stakeholder participants three of each (nurse managers, nurses and physicians) working at a regional hospital situated in the Northwest region of Cameroon. Inclusion criteria for the population was limited to qualified participants who work or are knowledgeable about corrupt business and management practices within a specific realm and an administrative level within the PHS. The sample for the study included a total of nine participants (three nurse managers, three nurses and three physicians) recruited using the purposive and convenience sampling method. The population and sample for this study was recruited by using the purposive and convenience sampling process. It involved searching and locating the personnel directory of the hospital system for names, contact information, position title and contacting participants by mail, email, and telephone until at least nine participants agreed to be interviewed.

Upon recruiting the required number of participants data collection commenced using semi-structured interviews in face-to-face sessions and in private offices or non-agency locations. For a multiple case study, Yin (2009) suggest a minimum of 6-10 interviews with six being the lowest number of interviews needed to achieve saturation. If saturation requirement was not met, recruitment would have continued until saturation requirement was achieved (Yin, 2009. As such, the researcher developed a total of nine open-ended interview questions, including three sub-questions. The research and interview questions were developed based on the study's problems and included several constructs such as (motives, interest, rationale, reasoning and problems) as descriptors of the term *perception*. Each interview was conducted and using a Samsung Galaxy Note 4 phone for recording. Also, a face-sheet and open and closing guide was used during the interview process. The face-sheet was used in recording circumstances of the interview, including date, location and time. Each interview lasted between 0-45 minutes. Participant responses were recorded during each interview and transcribed verbatim. In conducting the study Yin's (2009) organized was used in guiding the researcher. During the interview process, participant responses were recorded using a Samsung Galaxy phone and transcribed verbatim in a Word document to be saved in password-protected personal laptop only accessible by the researcher. While Yin's (2009) comprehensive steps was used in conducting the study Clarke and Braun's (2017) organized phases was used in analyzing the data.

The organized steps in the study included (a) refining the interview questions based at least three expert reviews and feedback in field tests, (b) participant recruitment, (c) conducting semi-structured interviews and taking written notes, and (d) using deductive thematic analysis in recursively searching, identifying and interpreting the data (Braun & Braun, 2017; Yin, 2009). The organized process of the thematic analysis included (a) recursively searching, familiarizing in taking notes and generating initial codes, (b) identifying themes and sub-themes, (c) reviewing and defining similar themes and (d) naming and describing participant perceptions of the phenomena in relation to the research questions (Clarke & Braun, 2017; Yin, 2009). The study had a main assumption, as well as limitation and delimitation.

The main assumption of this study was that the selected research method qualitative, multiple case study with semi-structured interviews was best for the study as it allowed the researcher in eliciting and yielding relevant stakeholder perceptions about the corruptive business and management practices in the PHS and measures in diminishing it. A potential limitation for this study was that of bias as participants may not be truthful and honest with their responses because of sensitivities in discussing a topic like corruption and thus, affecting external validity in generalizing the findings. This limitation was overcome by scheduling face-to-face interviews in the private offices of participants and private locations where appropriate.

A delimitation in research studies are the established boundaries or aspects of the study that the researcher can control (Davis, 2013). The geographic setting of the study, the qualitative, multiple case study method and the convenience, the selected participants and purposive sampling process were the established boundaries of this study (Davis, 2013). The study investigated the perceptions of key stakeholders who work or have knowledge about corrupt business and management practices in the PHS of Cameroon. The researcher also used an informed consent form in ensuring participants are aware of their right to voluntarily participate and to end their participation at any time. Participants were required to sign, scan and email or mail back the consent form as a requirement for participating.

Chapter 4

Findings

This section contains the themes and subthemes that resulted from the deductive thematic analysis of the data, including the direct quotations from participants. The results are presented within the context of the research questions. This section begins with the interview results with each research question, a table of the themes and subthemes, and the direct responses of participants. While Clark and Braun's (2017) organized steps guided the analysis, Yin's (2013a) framework analysis of case study units and sub-units initiated the thematic analyses of each individual unit (each stakeholder), each sub-unit (comprising two or more stakeholders) and the sample as a whole (comprising all nine stakeholders in order to achieve construct validity), as well as the thematic analyses of the relationships between the units and sub-units. The results of the analysis were presented per each research question.

RQ1. How do PHS stakeholders perceive corrupt business and management practices of bribing before receiving better care in a health care facility, unjustified absences, and tardiness while being paid, maintaining a "nice" position and promoting the hiring of family members in the PHS of Cameroon?

Table 1 provides a summary of the themes and subthemes from stakeholder responses to RQ1. Deductive thematic analysis of the responses to the question resulted in the identification of two themes: (a) Mismanagement, and (b) High Unemployment. Deductive analysis of the responses also

85

resulted in the identification of three subthemes: (a) motivation, (b) low compensation, and (c) staff shortage. The results answered the research question as to stakeholders' perceptions, views, opinions, and understandings about corruption within the PHS of Cameroon. Stakeholders overtly discussed the failures of management and lack of leadership in developing rules and processes design to mitigate corrupt practices within the hospital system.

Table 1: Stakeholders' Perceptions of Corruption

Number	Theme	Subtheme
1	Mismanagement	Motivation
		Low Compensation
		Staff Shortage
2	High Unemployment	

Theme 1: Mismanagement. The theme, mismanagement was converged as the overarching perception of corruption because seven participants (P1, P2, P3, P4, P6, P7, P8, and P9) indicated that management had failed to put in place rules and processes to mitigate corruptive practices relating to treatment of patients, staff/client relationships and the hiring and promotion of staff members. The participants also mentioned impunity as major factor in the existence of corruption as staff members who are reported for corrupt activities and poor performance are not disciplined and held accountable. Seven out of nine participants affirmed organizational policies and rules on preventing corruption were either non-existent or outdated. They also stated that when such policies exist, they are not properly communicated to staff members. For example, participant P1 converged that

86

"Management does not have an effective means of measuring daily staff performance," and/or output to ensure staff members are working and in achieving desired and "measurable results."

P1 affirmed that

No one is ever disciplined, punished and held accountable when employees do not follow institutional procedures and/or processes for handling patients while in the triage process and leading to patient neglect, queues and even dead.

Participant P2 concurred

When staff members are caught or reported for patient neglect, asking for a bribe as a condition for providing better service, and selling drugs to patients, they are not disciplined thus, giving employees a sense of "entitlement." Participant

Participant P7 affirmed

Insubordination among staff members and the failure of management to fix the problem is the main cause of corruption within the hospital system and it is appalling that it still exists.

Participant P8 affirmed

Because "rules and/or policies are not constantly updated and communicated to staff members" they are not aware of how to improve their level of service. While seven participants converged organizational mismanagement and accountability as contributing to corruption

Participant P5 mentioned that

"I am not sure about it." Specifically, there was construct validity in an individual stakeholder as well as administrative

87

stakeholder group level as seven participants from all three administrative realms mentioned mismanagement as contributing to corruption.

Subtheme 1: Motivation. The subtheme, motivation, was deemed because five participants (P1, P2, P3, P4, and P7) converged that management was not doing enough to motivate staff members, in terms of providing financial reward and expressing verbal appreciation when employees perform exceptionally well. The participants mentioned that a lack of motivation leads to low morale and a feeling that their work is not valued and thus, affects their attitudes and behaviors towards patients/clients and the organization. For example, participant P1 mentioned that

> Management should make it as part of their job to appreciate staff members when they do an excellent job, including providing financial reward and recognition. The absence of appreciation the participant acknowledged leads to low staff morale and affects job output. In addition, the participant stated that, when staff members do more and are not financially rewarded, they resort to taking bribe as a reward for "working extra hard."

Participant P7 affirmed

"An employee who is not fully motivated socially and financially will be vulnerable to corruption," However, while participant P7 stated a lack of motivation as a rationale for engaging in corrupt activities, the participant acknowledged that corruption within the hospital cannot solely be placed on a lack of motivation as there exists some form of motivation in every unit; although "it is very small." According to the participant, staff corruption may be a problem of "staff/patient influence." The participant mentioned that patients and care givers "influence nurses' attitudes to provide extra services through financial persuasion in order to concentrate more on the patient." In such a situation, "nurses are left with no option but to comply given the lack of financial and emotional motivation they already have about the agency." Additionally, the participant stated that patients pay bribes so as "not to wait in a queue" even when a staff member is not asking for it.

Subtheme 2: Low Compensation. The subtheme, low compensation, was converged because five participants (P1, P3, P6, P7, and P8) mentioned that personnel salaries were very low and management, including the government is not taking steps to increase it. For example, participant P1 mentioned that

Salaries are very "low" and "cannot support your daily upkeep." Because of this "employees engage in dubious ways of making money as an option."

Participant P3 affirmed

Employees engage in corruption because salaries and/or pay are "very low compared to the private sector." The participant further mentioned that because of low salaries, it creates a feeling of "dissatisfaction" thus, "affecting staff attitudes and behavior towards work and clients." However, the participant did strike an assuaging tone about some efforts "one could say very minor" by management in mitigating corruption by stating that "In all, am grateful for my institution." "They are working hard to curb such practices."

Participant P6 concurred

Nurses may be tempted to take bribes from patients or carers (those who care for patients) because of low salaries.

Subtheme 3: Staff Shortage. Deductive analysis of the responses to the RQ1 resulted in the identification of the subtheme, staff shortage. The subtheme, staff shortage, was converged because six participants (P1, P2, P3, P4, P6, and P8) responded that there is an acute shortage of staff as well as qualified personnel given the number of patients served.

Participant P3, for instance, converged that
Due to acute staff shortage, "nurses are required to take care of more patients than they can handle," leading to patient queue and neglect. To remedy their situation, "patients pay bribes to get the nurses' attention."

Participant P4 affirmed
"Less staff on duty will play a role because at times you see one nurse on duty for about 20-30 patients." In such a scenario, the "carers" (family members who care for loved ones while in a hospital) "will look for a way that the nurse will pay particular or special attention to his or her patient."

Theme 2: High Unemployment. Deductive thematic analysis of participant responses to RQ1 resulted to the theme, high unemployment. The theme, high unemployment was deemed because five participants (P2, P3, P4, P7, and P8) converged that high unemployment in Cameroon was a rationale for corruption. For example, participant P4 responded that employees pay bribes to superiors to maintain a job because "we are in a country or region where unemployment is a serious problem." Getting a job in Cameroon is very difficult. In such a situation, "those who manage to get into the system prefer to stay even after retirement." As such, this must only prevail if you bribe a superior to "maintain your job" as well as promoted.

Participant P8 affirmed

"Asking for bribes before providing services is morally wrong" and has no place in an institution devoted to caring for a vulnerable population. The participant further stated that because jobs are hard to find, "employees will do whatever to maintain their jobs" and thus, will pay a bribe to superiors to maintain a job and not be transferred to a rural area. Specifically, there was construct validity in an individual level and administrative realm level as five participants from all three administrative realms affirmed that high unemployment was a factor in corruption.

RQ1a. How do PHS stakeholders perceive other forms of corrupt business and management practices that exist in the PHS of Cameroon?

Table 2: Stakeholders Perceptions of the Different Forms of Corruption

Number	Theme	Subtheme
1	Diversion	
2	Extortion	
3	Embezzlement	

Table 2 above provides a summary of the themes and subtheme from stakeholder responses to RQ1a. Deductive thematic analysis of the responses to the question resulted in the identification of three themes: (a) Diversion, (b) Extortion, and (c) Embezzlement. The results answered the research question as to stakeholders' perceptions, views, opinions, and understandings of other forms of corruption within the PHS of Cameroon.

Theme 1: Diversion. The theme, diversion, was determined after thematic deductive analysis of participant responses to RQ1a. The theme, diversion, was identified because five participants (P1, P2, P4, P6, and P7) responded that staff members and specifically, physicians, regularly divert patients to private hospitals in which they have a direct financial interest. For example, participant P1 mentioned that

During consultations, physicians routinely deviate patients from public hospitals to private clinics or hospitals where they work. "They send patients there for examinations/ investigations, follow-ups and consultations." The participant also stated that health technicians (laboratory technicians, physiotherapists, dental engineers) and some medical specialists, including surgeons, gynecologists, and orthodontists) conduct private practice in the hospital; "In this practice, the individual collects money from the client directly while rendering the service; however, the institution (hospital) has no formal record of the service(s) rendered" as well as the money paid.

Participant P4 affirmed

Some physicians refer patients to perform lab tests and see a specialist in a private hospital after seeing the patient in the public hospital.

Participant P6 affirmed

Staff members often divert funds from the "special motivation" program which was implemented in every unit and/or department. Employees routinely participate in special motivation fund from their units while also participate in general staff motivation of the hospital system. The authorities and staffs of such units claim they generate the money; however, consider this scenario "a patient is consulted, hospitalized, does lab exams and buy drugs. The staff of the lab and pharmacy were motivated because much money was spent by the patient." However, "the consultants and the nurses in the wards were not." While five participants affirmed the occurrence of diversion,

Participant P3 responded that
I am not aware of any form of diversion.

Participant 5 affirmed
Not aware of any form of corruption

Participants P8 concurred by stating that
I have not come across such activities within the hospital system. Specifically, there was individual and inter-group construct validity as five participants from two separate stakeholder administrative realms affirmed the existence of diversion.

Theme 2: Extortion. The theme, extortion, was identified after a deductive analysis of participant responses to RQ1. The theme was deemed because six participants (P1, P2, P3, P4, P6, and P8) mentioned that staff members use their position to extort money from patients and/or clients. For example,

Participant P1 stated that
Nurses and physicians condition the type of care they provide to a client based on the level of patronage they receive. The participant also stated that physicians maintain a "small pharmacy" of essential drugs in their offices for sale to clients. The participant further mentioned that managers "unfairly divide the proceeds giving to each department for motivating staff members by taking into consideration his/her personal relationship with the staff rather than productivity as prescribed by hospital guidelines." According to the participant, such practices lead to an

uncomfortable work environment between personnel and management as well as personnel and clients thus, hampering job "satisfaction and the credibility of the institution."

Participant P2 affirmed

Recently, extortion has been the most rampant form of corruption in the hospital. "Demanding patients to pay more for services than they are required to." The extra money goes into the staffs' pocket, leaving the patient impoverished and unable to foot the hospital bills. A good example is asking a "pregnant woman to pay 150,000 frs. CFA or ($266) for a C/S (Caesarean Section) which should normally cost 40,000 frs. CFA or ($71) as stipulated by the government." The participant added that "personally, the punitive measures for such acts should be increased and the public sensitized so that they don't fall prey to such vandals."

Participants P4 affirmed

Some nurses routinely ask for bribes before directing clients on where they need to go and see a certain doctor and/or show them the unit they need to go for service. Though seven participants affirmed extortion as another form of corruption that exists within the hospital system, two participants (P5 and P7) did not affirm its existence. For example,

Participant P5 affirmed
"I can't tell."

Participant P7 converged that
"I don't know of other forms of corrupt business and management practices."

Theme 3: Embezzlement. The theme, embezzlement, was deemed because three participants (P1, P2, and P7) converged that staff members in high positions routinely embezzle funds that have been earmarked for infrastructure improvement and buying much-needed equipment. For instance, participant P2 stated that

Top-level hospital officials who are charged with executing infrastructure improvements and procurement of vital hospital supplies embezzle funds appropriated by the government by putting it into their pockets. Because of this, patients requiring specialized services have to seek care out of their area of residence in neighboring towns and at times out of Cameroon. Such costs in seeking treatment "is out of reach for most Cameroonians." The participant added that "I decry this ill (embezzlement) alongside all other corrupt activities in the hospital and I think the culprits should be brought to law."

Participant P7 affirmed

Embezzlement is a "major problem in this hospital, and I think it is morally and ethically wrong as it prevents the institution from performing its primary duty to the public, which is to provide care and safe lives."

RQ2. How do stakeholders perceive ways to diminish and improve the business and management practices that exist in the PHS of Cameroon?

Table 3 above provides a summary of the themes and subthemes from stakeholder responses to RQ2.

Table 3: Stakeholders Perceptions of Measures for Diminishing Corrupt Business and Management Practices

Number	Theme	Subtheme
1	Organizational Change	Motivation
		Empowerment
		Accountability
		Increase Compensation

Deductive thematic analysis of the responses to the question resulted in the identification of one theme: (a) Organizational Change. Deductive thematic analysis of the responses also resulted in four subthemes: (a) Motivation, (b) Empowerment, (c) Accountability, and (d) Increase Compensation. The results answered the research question as to stakeholders' perceptions of ways and measures in diminishing corrupt business and management practices within the PHS of Cameroon.

Theme 1: Organizational Change. Deductive thematic analysis of participant responses to RQ2 resulted in the identification of the organizational change as the main theme. The theme, organizational change, was converged because all nine participants mentioned that management and the government (Ministry of Public Health) should adopt several measures in order to diminish corrupt practices. The participants responded that upgrading hospital infrastructure, procuring essential equipment, hiring more staff, boosting staff morale through motivation, installing a strong anti-corruption panel with legal authority and involving staff members in the decision-making process as examples of ways in diminishing corrupt business and management practices. For example, participant P1 converged that

"The government should create (V.I.P) services in all big public hospitals," such service facilities should be created in "towns with populations of more than 500,000 inhabitants." According to the participant, V.I.P service facilities are important because "they tend to have all the requisite care services, including better-trained personnel and equipment thus, improving patient outcome, mitigate long queues, and bribes to receive better services." The participant further stated that management should boost employee morale by providing better working environment such as buying better equipment and upgrading antiquated infrastructure.

Participant P2 affirmed
"I will start by praising hospital authorities and the government for the various measures they have put in place to combat corruption in the hospital system." Although the ideas are brilliant; however, "in the context of my country most of these measures end only on papers and in managements' offices." For example, "in the last decade or more, the number of people brought to law nationwide for corrupt practices in hospitals can be counted with our fingertips." The participant also stated that

"People listen to public service announcements about corruption but, keep-up with such practices, since they know all the repeated announcements are propaganda. Deep down inside them, they say with much conviction that they will never be arrested." According to the participant, management and the government needs to take some steps to demonstrate its seriousness in fighting corruption within the hospital. As such, the participant mentioned that

"I think to diminish corruption in the PHS, a change of mentality has to be the first measure to be put in place. From basic education, our children and citizens have to be trained on the values of nation building. Most of the sectors in our country are corrupt, as such, it is but normal that it has creeped very fast into the hospital system." "I will conclude here by saying that the government needs to demonstrate its seriousness by bringing more people to the law. As such the public will sit up thereby reducing these ills of corruption in hospitals."

Participant P3 confirmed

Management should hire more staff to reduce the patient/staff ratio and workload thus, improve quality of care.

Participant P4 affirmed

"Though the various anti-corruption actions taken by management are applaudable; however, they don't go far enough. According to the participant "more needs to be done as it has reduced corruption somewhat; however, people still look for ways to engage in corrupt activities." Specifically, there was construct validity in both individual and administrative group level as all nine participants from each administrative realm affirmed organizational change as a measure in diminishing corruption.

Participant P8 confirmed

"Decentralize the management of hospital functions and involve heads of units and chief of services (who should be qualified personnel within their respective departments in the decision-making process)."

Subtheme 1: Motivation. Deductive analysis of participant responses to RQ1 resulted to the identification of the subtheme recognition. The subtheme, motivation, was converged because eight participants (P1, P2, P3, P5, P6, P7, P8, and P9) indicated that management is not doing a better job in motivating staff members when they do an excellent job. In particular, the participants mentioned that staff motivation, including recognition for job excellence, is not currently a policy of the hospital and should be considered by management to show their appreciation for working hard. For example, participant P1 stated that

"Management should boost personnel morale by ensuring both unit and hospital-wide motivation pay is prompt and fair."

Participant P2 affirmed
"Motivating employees and specifically members of the anti-corruption committee in the hospital will spur and push them to perform their duty with due diligence. When this is done workers in most hospitals will sit-up because they will be scared to be brought to the law."

Participant P7 affirmed
"Management should properly and consistently motivate staffs for their efforts.

Subtheme 2: Empowerment. The subtheme, empowerment, was deemed because five participants (P1, P2, P3, P6, and P9) responded that management should implement an awareness and education program designed to educate and empower clients about their rights while in the hospital in order to reduce corruption. For instance, Participant P1 mentioned that

"Management should also empower peripheral administrators, including unit heads and ward charges by giving them authority to take disciplinary actions on subordinates for lateness, absenteeism and other malign behaviors"

Participant P3 affirmed

"Management should also educate clients and/or patients about their right to receive services without paying bribes, including the cost of each service and procedure as mandated by the government."

Participant P6 affirmed

"Educating clients is critical in reducing corruption."

Participant P9 affirmed

"Information is the base for reducing corruption within the structure." According to the participant "when people are informed, even things that look like a corruption, will appear differently."

Subtheme 3: Accountability. Deductive thematic analysis of participant responses to RQ2 resulted in the identification of the subtheme accountability. The subtheme, accountability, was deemed because seven participants (P1, P2, P3, P6, P7, P8, and P9) reported that management and the government need to implement a system of accountability such as audit control, strong anti-corruption panel and severe punishment if they are serious in mitigating corruption. For instance, participant P1 reported that

"The government should adopt legislation that seek to sanction and penalize authorities who effectuate employment to family and/or friends without prior publicity of the vacancy." According to the participant, when positions become available, "recruitment must be conducted by a panel of at least five persons, excluding the vote holder with direct supervision of the members." The participant further stated that; "staff guilty of patient deviation, parallel sales of drugs, conducting private practice within and outside the facility should be severely punished financially and even judicially."

Participant P2 affirmed

"Though the installation of anti-corruption bodies is working well in certain hospitals; however, the majority of those in charge of running these bodies often do not do so. Because of this, the personnel feel free to continue with such practices." According to the participant, "anti-corruption bodies should prove to the citizens that they are not toothless bulldogs." "A few arrests and corrective measures here and there will make most corrupt employees think twice before getting involved in corrupt acts."

Participant P3 acknowledged

"Management should step up punishment for corrupt behavior for both nurses/clients."

Participant P6 confirmed

Management should take several steps to diminish corrupt practices namely: (a) put information on notice boards concerning the wrong doings of the staff, (b) make available the phone numbers of anti-corruption officials to facilitate reporting of corrupt activities by clients and other staff members, (c) install cameras in unit wards and other high corruption service areas, and (d) setup disciplinary council to punish corrupters.

Participant P7 affirmed

"Anti-corruption committees should be setup in all units to monitor and punish corrupt activities."

Participant P8 affirmed

"From my point of view, most if not all of these measures put in place to diminish corruption have been between the borderline of ineffectiveness and failure." "Most often, the system of audit is absent and even when applicable, such auditors themselves are easily corrupted (popular opinion)." The participant stated that "I stand by this opinion because the evidence is clear." "Take the example of our hospital, look at the rate of growth in terms of infrastructure and degradation of equipment despite the amount of income generated and government subvention."

Participant P9 affirmed

"Setup strong audit control system both internally and externally and ensure checks and balances between the bodies." Specifically, there was construct validity both individually and stakeholder group as seven participants from all administrative realms affirmed accountability as a measure for diminishing corrupt business and management practices within the hospital system.

Subtheme 4: Increase Compensation. The subtheme, increase compensation, was converged because six participants (P1, P2, P3, P5, P6, and P8) converged that management and the government should increase employee pay/salary in order to boost morale and reduce the need for employees to engage in corrupt activities. For example, participant P1 indicated that

"Salaries should be increase taking into consideration market prices and harmonized across the public sector."

Participant P2 affirmed

"An increase in salary and the motivation of health personnel will greatly reduce corruption because there are many individuals who involve themselves in these practices in order to make ends meet."

Participants P3 affirmed

The government and management should pay more and provide adequate payment packages to employees.

Participant P5 confirmed

Adequate payment packages need to be provided

Participant P6 concurred

Management needs to provide good payment package for staff

Participant P8 affirmed

The government should "increase wages for hospital staff (administrators, doctors, nurses, lab techs etc.)."

Evaluation of the Findings

The purpose of this qualitative, multiple case study was to provide further understanding of how to diminish corrupt business and management practices that continue to lead to increased monetary cost to individuals and delays in seeking preventative care within the PHS of Cameroon (Kankeu et al., 2016; Kankeu & Ventelou, 2016; Tinyami et al., 2015; Yamb & Bayemi, 2017). As such, the qualitative, multiple case study with semi-structured interviews was used to investigate the perceptions, views, and understandings of a diverse group of stakeholders, including nurse managers, nurses, and physicians of how to diminish corrupt business and management practices within the hospital system. The researcher used stakeholder theory in understanding and explaining the views and perceptions of stakeholders about their interest in corruption, rationale or justification for corruption and the measures in diminishing it (Freeman, 1984; 2011). This section contains the evaluation of the findings and was presented per each research question and its resulting themes and subthemes.

RQ1. How do PHS stakeholders perceive corrupt business and management practices of bribing before receiving better care in a health care facility, unjustified absences, tardiness while being paid, maintaining a "nice" position, and promoting the hiring of family members in the PHS of Cameroon?

Theme 1 Mismanagement. The theme, mismanagement, was identified based on participant responses that management had failed in its core responsibilities to put in place rules and policies to mitigate corruptive practices in relation to the treatment of patients, measuring daily output performance, impunity and transparency in the hiring and promotion of staff members. According to stakeholder normative principle, management's key responsibilities involves balancing competing interest and giving equal consideration to all stakeholder claims in terms of implementing rules and processes that is fair and transparent to all stakeholders (Donaldson & Preston, 1995; Freeman, 1984).

Consistent with stakeholder theory, the finding that PHS managers have failed to ensure that its policies for recruitment and hiring new employees are fair and transparent, rules for treating patients in the triage are frequently updated and effectively communicated, impunity is checked, and staff daily performance are measured to enhance efficiency were to be expected (Freeman, 1984; Purnell & Freeman, 2012). In line with the findings, Brady and Davies (2014) revealed that project failures, including cost overruns and delays within project management settings such as hospitals and information

104

technology depend on how effective project managers can effectively ensure processes and rules for properly identifying key stakeholder competencies are followed to enhance project success. Brady and Davies' (2014) contention was affirmed by participant P1 that rules and processes for treating patients in triage are "outdated" and not followed leading to "patient neglect and even death." Similarly, Harrison et al (2015) affirmed that an agency that manages for its stakeholders ensures its survivability and success. As such, the theme, mismanagement, was to be expected given the corruption in the hospital system.

Within the context of the current literature, Hope (2014) revealed that corruption within public hospitals in Kenya are a result of a culture of corruption due to mismanagement, including a lack of accountability and impunity. Thus, the theme, mismanagement was to be expected as seven out of nine participants perceived that employees are not severely punished when reported for corruption and that no policy exists to measure daily performance. The findings also supported the study of Kankeu et al.; (2016) in which employees demand bribes from patients to avoid being in a queue and receive better care services. Whereas, Tinyami et al.; (2015) revealed that employees made payments to managers to maintain a "juicy" position and avoid being transferred to rural areas, the findings revealed that employees pay bribes to managers to obtain and maintain their positions because securing and maintaining a job in Cameroon is very difficult due to the high rate of unemployment. As such, the finding was not expected.

Subtheme 1: Motivation. The subtheme, motivation, was deemed because participants converged that hospital managers were not doing enough to motivate staff members, in terms of providing financial reward and expressing verbal appreciation thus, affecting employee attitudes and behavior towards clients and the organization. Participant P2, for instance, perceived that an employee who is not socially and financially motivated may be tempted to engage in corruption. From a normative stakeholder perspective, scholars (Freeman et al., 2007; Tantalo & Priem, 2014) contended that when managers are responsive to stakeholder demands, it enhances stakeholder collaboration and increases agency value and performance. Brady and Davies (2014) affirmed that when project managers provide consistent motivation, including providing financial incentives and recognition, it results to project success, including cost savings due to early project completion. King (2015) contend that agency decisions should consider the interest of all stakeholders by engaging and responding to their demands. As such, the subtheme, motivation, was to be expected given the corruption where participants perceived that management is not doing enough to consistently provide financial motivation to staff members and affects their morale thus, attitudes to clients (Freeman et al. 2007; Tantalo & Priem, 2014). However, the revelation by participant P8 that staff/client influence rather than only motivation was a rationale for stakeholder engagement in accepting bribes was unexpected.

Within the context of the current literature, the findings that management has failed in consistently provide verbal and financial reward to motivate staff members for exceptional job performance was expected given the findings by Yamb and Bayemi (2017) that revealed corruption within public hospitals in the Littoral Region of Cameroon was due to a lack of motivation and suggested that hospital managers should consider providing financial motivation to enhance satisfaction and reduce corruption.

Subtheme 2: Low Compensation. The subtheme, low compensation, was identified because participants mentioned that personnel salaries were very low as management and the government are not taking steps to increase it. Because of this, employees engage in dubious ways of making money to provide for upkeep. Participant P6, for example, revealed employees are

106

tempted to take bribes from patients or carers because of low salaries. Otherwise, there was no discussion on low compensation perspectives and organizational function with regards to stakeholder understanding. Thus, the findings may be seen as a contribution to stakeholder theory.

As such, the findings may be viewed as a new construct (a contribution) for stakeholder theory.

Within the context of the current study, the findings that salaries/pay are too low and leading to employees engaging in corrupt activities to maintain their upkeep was to be expected and was consistent with Yamb and Bayemi (2017) that revealed corruption in public hospital within public hospitals in the Littoral Region of Cameroon was because of the low pay of civil servants. Similarly, Kagotho, Bunger, and Wagner (2016) contend that corruption within public hospitals in Kenya was due to the low levels of civil servant pay. Also, An and Kweon (2017) revealed that increasing wages for public employees resulted in low-levels of corruption especially in developing countries such as Cameroon and Nigeria so that statements by five participants (P2, P3, P4, P7, and P8) that employees accept bribes and leave work early to work in other part-time job to augment their pay was to be expected.

Subtheme 3: Staff Shortage. The subtheme, staff shortage, was deemed based on participant responses that there is an acute shortage of staff and qualified personnel given the number of clients served and management has failed to address the problem. The findings also revealed that at times there is one nurse on duty in support of 20-30 clients and leading to staff exhaustion and clients offering bribes to get special attention even when the nurse is not asking for it. Otherwise, there was no discussion on staff shortage perspectives and organizational function with regards to stakeholder understanding. Thus, the findings may be seen as a contribution to stakeholder theory.

107

Within the context of current scholarly literature, whereas author Kankeu et al., (2016) revealed that family members and patients make bribe payments to nurses as a condition for accessing and receiving better treatment and care services. However, the findings revealed that because of acute staff shortage, clients and their carers offer bribes to nurses when they are not asking for it in order to receive particular or special attention from the nurse was a new revelation and contributed to current literature.

Theme 2: High Unemployment. The theme, high unemployment was identified based on participant responses that finding a job in Cameroon is very difficult due to the high rate of unemployment. Because of this, those who manage to get into the system pay a bribe to maintain their position. Otherwise, there was no discussion on high unemployment perspectives and organizational function with regards to stakeholder understanding. Thus, the finding may be seen as a contribution to stakeholder theory. In previous research Yamb and Bayemi (2017) revealed that doctors and other staff members pay bribes to superiors to avoid being transferred to rural areas and maintaining a "nice" position so that the results would have been expected; however, the findings that paying bribes to maintain a "nice" position was because of the high rate of unemployment in Cameroon was a new finding.

RQ1a. How do PHS stakeholders perceive other forms of corrupt business and management practices that exist in the PHS of Cameroon?

Thematic deductive analysis of participant responses resulted in the identification of three themes and includes the following: (a) diversion, (b) extortion, and (c) embezzlement.

Theme 1 Diversion. The theme, diversion, was determined based on participant responses that staff members and specifically physicians and health specialists regularly divert patients to private hospitals in which they have a direct financial interest after seeing clients in their office. In the practice of diversion, the physician or staff send patients for examinations/investigations, follow-ups and consultations. A second form of diversion occurs where health technicians (laboratory technicians, physiotherapists, dental engineers) and some medical specialists, including surgeons, gynecologists, and orthodontists) conduct private practice in the hospital. In this practice, the staff member collects money from the client directly while rendering the service; however, the institution (hospital) has no formal record of the service(s) being provided and the money paid. Otherwise, there was no discussion on diversion perspectives and organizational function with regards to stakeholder understanding. Thus, the findings may be seen as a contribution to stakeholder theory. Within the context of current scholarly literature and the current study, participant perceptions of diversion as a form of corruption has not received attention. As such, the findings may be regarded as a contribution to current scholarship.

Theme 2 Extortion. The theme, extortion, was identified after a deductive analysis of participant responses to RQ1. The theme was deemed because six participants (P1, P2, P3, P4, P6, and P8) out of nine mentioned that staff members use their position to extort money from patients. In this form of corruption, nurses and physicians condition the type of care they provide to a client based on the level of patronage they receive. A second form of extortion occurs where physicians maintain a mini pharmacy of essential drugs in their offices for sale to clients. A third form of extortion occurs where managers unfairly divide the proceeds giving to each department for motivating staff members by taking into consideration his/her personal relationship with the staff rather than productivity as prescribed by hospital guidelines. Otherwise, there was no discussion on extortion perspectives and organizational function with regards to stakeholder understanding. As such, the findings might be considered a contribution for stakeholder theory.

In previous research Kankeu et al.; (2016) revealed that hospital staff members illegally keep and sell drugs, including anti-retroviral drugs such as the Human Immune Virus and Acquired Immune Deficiency Syndrome which are supposed to be free to patients. Similarly, Yamb and Bayemi (2017) revealed that employees in public hospitals within the Littoral province sell drugs to patients that are supposed to be free. These studies supported the findings that physicians operate a mini pharmacy in their office for sale to clients. However, the findings that medical specialists such as gynecologists extort money from expectant mothers by charging $266 for a C/S (Caesarean Section) instead of $71 as stipulated by the government was not expected.

Theme 3: Embezzlement. The theme, embezzlement, was identified based on participant responses that top-level managers routinely embezzle funds earmarked for maintaining and upgrading hospital infrastructure and equipment. According to stakeholder normative principle, management's core actions and responsibilities should be on the agency and its stakeholders and from the stakeholders to the agency for enhancing value creation and agency success (Donaldson & Preston, 1995; Freeman, 1984; Tantalo & Priem, 2014). Tantalo and Priem (2014) observed that when management's actions affect another stakeholder, it prevents effective stakeholder collaboration and reduces value creation for all stakeholders. Thus, statements by participant P2 that because of embezzlement by top managers "patients requiring specialized services have to seek care out of their area of residence in neighboring towns and at times out of Cameroon supported those of Tantalo and Priem (2014) as it

110

affects the PHS' stakeholders (citizens of Cameroon) by resulting to increased monetary costs in seeking care services.

Within the context of current scholarly literature, the findings that top managers embezzle hospital funds meant for infrastructure improvements were consistent with the study by Agbiboa (2012) that revealed management level corruption in the form of embezzlement in Nigeria. Similarly, Njong and Ngantcha (2013) revealed management level corruption within the health care delivery chain in Cameroon where hospital officials abuse funds meant for buying supplies. Equally, Osifo (2014) affirmed corruption by top managers within public hospitals in Nigeria and Cameroon so that the findings that top managers within the PHS embezzle funds was expected.

RQ2. How do stakeholders perceive ways to diminish and improve the business and management practices that exists in the PHS of Cameroon?

Thematic deductive analysis of participant responses to RQ2 resulted in the identification of the theme, organizational change (motivation, empowerment, accountability, and increase compensation.

Theme 1 Organizational Change. The theme, organizational change, was identified because all nine participants mentioned that in order to reduce and mitigate corruptive business and management practices, hospital managers and the government (Ministry of Public Health) should adopt several policies, rules, and regulations, including strengthening anti-corruption bodies, installing an internal and external audit board, streamline decision-making processes to engage key stakeholders, empower denizens, and increase compensation. According to stakeholder strategic management practices for success, stakeholder theorists (Gupta & Sharma,

111

2014) contend that when good governance practices consisting a combination of policies, rules, laws on ways to manage an agency such as, stakeholder engagement, proper internal audit controls requirements, and an independent management board, it led to improved agency performance and success of Indian and South Korean firms (Gupta & Sharma, 2014).

In line with this argument, Ayuso et al.; (2014) revealed a significant and positive relationship between a firm's internal audit board processes, including its financial disclosure records and increase in level of confidence among stakeholders leading to a high degree of trust among investors. As such, the findings that PHS managers should implement internal and external audit boards to increase financial transparency to mitigate corruption was expected. Consistent with the findings that PHS managers should decentralize management processes to include and engage key stakeholders in the decision-making process, Brady and Davies (2014) Eskerod et al.; (2015) argued that when stakeholders are not properly engaged in agency decision-making processes, the potential for project failure increases. Similarly, King (2015) contend that agency decisions should consider the interest of all stakeholders by engaging and soliciting their opinions.

Other stakeholder theorists (Pandi-Perumal et al., 2015; Starks et al., 2015) have suggested stakeholder engagement as a management practice that seek to involve stakeholders in a "positive manner" in all aspects involving organizational actions to enhance success. Starks et al. (2015), for example, revealed that when key stakeholders were involved in the decision-making process of creating treatment programs for depression within Indian reservations in the state of Alaska, it resulted in the creation of early detection programs for diagnosing depression and reduction in depression among young adults. Notwithstanding the expectations of the findings, the revelation by participant P1 management and the government should

112

create V.I.P health facilities in towns with populations of more than 500,000 inhabitants to improve quality of care, reduce costs to clients and prevent corruption in bribes in order to receive better care service and hire more staff to increase patient/staff ratio to reduce patient queue and corruption were not expected.

In line with the current scholarly literature, Agbiboa (2012) suggested the need for government and civil service managers to create and strengthen anti-corruption bodies as a measure for reducing widespread corruption in the Nigerian public sector. Similarly, Hope (2014) affirmed the creation of strong anti-corruption bodies that are anchored in sound legal systems for reducing corruption within Kenyan public hospital. Thus, the revelation that PHS managers and the government should create and strengthen anti-corruption bodies to investigate and punish corrupt employees was expected. However, the findings as perceived by participant P8 that PHS managers should "decentralize the management of hospital functions and involve heads of units and chief of services (who should be qualified personnel within their respective departments in the decision-making process to reduce corruption)" was unexpected.

Subtheme 1: Motivation. As with the theme, organizational change, the subtheme, motivation, was deemed because eight out of nine participants (P1, P2, P3, P5, P6, P7, P8, and P9) converged that management should adopt and implement policies that seek to consistently provide financial and verbal motivation, including personal recognition to staff members when they do an excellent job to boost morale and increase worker attitudes and behaviors towards clients and the agency. Stakeholder management responsibilities involve balancing competing interests in terms of adopting and implementing policies, including providing financial incentives and recognition for exceptional service in a way that creates value for all stakeholders and ensures the survival of the agency (Donaldson & Preston, 1995; Freeman, 1984). Within stakeholder project management settings such as engineering and hospitals that have several departments, including unit and department heads, Brady and Davies (2014) revealed that when project managers implemented employee motivation programs, including providing financial incentives, it resulted to increased job satisfaction rates and led to early project completion rates and cost savings. As such, the findings that PHS managers should adopt and implement policies design to provide consistent financial and verbal motivation to boost morale was expected.

Consistent with current scholarly scholarship, Yamb and Bayemi (2017) revealed that corruption within public hospitals in Douala Cameroon was a result of lack of staff motivation by management and suggested that in order to reduce corruption, hospital managers and the government of Cameroon should consider policies to motivate staff members in order to reduce corruption. Agbiboa (2012) suggested that providing motivational incentives may help in reducing public corruption in Nigeria. Similarly, Kagotho et al. (2016) suggested that providing financial motivation may increase public sector worker morale in Kenya and reduce corruption. These contentions are in line with the findings of the current study as statements by participants (P2 and P7) that managers should consistently motivate staffs for their efforts and specifically anti-corruption employees to spur them to do their jobs with due diligence were expected.

Subtheme 2: Empowerment. The subtheme, empowerment, was identified based on participant statements that management and the government should implement policies design to empower unit heads and ward charges to take disciplinary actions on corruption within their departments to reduce corruption and educative programs design to sensitize the public about the ills of corruption, including their rights while receiving care services in health facilities. Otherwise, there was no discussion on

114

empowerment perspectives and organizational change with regards to stakeholder understanding.

Within the context of current literature, the findings were consistent with Walton and Peiffer (2017) that revealed education base corruptive programs can positively influence the public's assessment of corrupt practices in public institutions as educated individuals are more likely to report corrupt activities to authorities than less educated ones, thus diminishing its likelihood of occurring. Similarly, Fortunato and Panizza (2015) revealed a significant relationship between levels of education and good governance practices. Chidi (2014) contended that education-based corruption programs enable individuals to have an awareness and interest in ensuring that best business practices, including merit-based selection, hiring and promotion policies are strictly enforced thus, leading to less corruption. Aside from these studies, there was no discussion of perceived empowerment as a measure for diminishing corruptive business and management practices within the context of stakeholder theory. Thus, the theme, empowerment can be seen as a new construct (a contribution) to stakeholder theory.

Subtheme 3: Accountability. As with the theme organizational change, participant responses to the research question resulted in the identification of the subtheme accountability. The subtheme, accountability, was deemed because seven (P1, P2, P3, P6, P7, P8, and P9) out of nine participants reported that management and the government need to implement a system of accountability, including internal and external audit board control and strong anti-corruption committees in all units with authority to investigate and punish corrupt practices. Consistent with stakeholder strategic management practices for firm success, Ayuso et al. (2014) revealed a significant and positive relationship between a firm's audit board processes, including its financial disclosure records and increase in the level of confidence among stakeholders and leading to a high degree of

115

trust among investors. Similarly, Chan et al.; (2014) affirmed that agencies that consistently apply good governance practices, including independent audit boards and proper financial disclosure information as a management strategy are more likely to enhance their performance and value creation for its stakeholders than those that do not.

Within the context of the current scholarly literature and as with the theme organizational change, the findings that managers should implement anti-corruption committees in all units to investigate and punish corrupt practices supported the findings of Agbiboa (2012) in which he suggested the need for government and civil service managers to create and strengthen anti-corruption bodies as a measure for reducing widespread corruption in Nigerian public sector. In line with this contention, Hope (2014) affirmed the creation of strong anti-corruption bodies that are anchored in sound legal systems for reducing corruption within Kenyan public hospital. However, the findings as perceived by participant P6 about the specific measures that anti-corruption committees should consider to diminish corruption namely: (a) put information on notice boards concerning the wrong doings of the staff, (b) make available the phone numbers of anti-corruption officials to facilitate reporting of corrupt activities by clients and other staff members, and (c) install cameras in unit wards and other high corruption service areas were unexpected.

Subtheme 4: Increase Compensation. The subtheme, increase compensation, was converged based on participant responses that management and the government should increase employee pay/salary taking into consideration market prices and harmonized across the public sector in order to boost morale and reduce the need for employees to engage in corrupt activities. The findings also revealed that the government should provide adequate pay/salary packages to staff. Otherwise, there was no discussion on increase compensation perspectives and organizational change with regards to stakeholder understanding. The findings may also be seen as a contribution (a construct) for stakeholder theory.

Within the context of the current literature, the findings that management should increase employee salaries/pay is consistent with Yamb and Bayemi's (2017) suggestion in order reduce corruption within public hospitals in the Littoral Region of Cameroon, the government should increase civil servant salaries/pay. Similarly, Kagotho et al.; (2016) suggested that to reduce public sector corruption in Kenya, the government should increase public employee pay. An and Kweon (2017) further contend that increasing wages for public employees results in low-levels of corruption especially in developing countries such as Cameroon and Nigeria and Kenya. As such, the findings were expected.

Summary

The data collection process consisted of three semi-structured open-ended questions through telephone in the private offices of participants where appropriate. Each interview was recorded and transcribed verbatim into a Microsoft Word document and saved in a password enabled personal laptop. The transcribed data went through a recursive process of manual analysis and using Braun and Clarks' (2017) organized steps as discussed in chapter three.

Within the context of the results, stakeholder responses to RQ1 revealed that stakeholder rationale for corruption was due to mismanagement. Participants perceived that management had failed in consistently reward and motivate personnel, provide better pay/salary and hire more staff to reduce exhaustion. With regards to RQ1a, participants perceived other corrupt business and management practices in diversion, extortion and embezzlement by physicians, specialists, and lab technicians.

The implication of these corrupt practices is that it affects the ability of the PHS to efficiently manage and deliver on its core mission of improving and delivering better healthcare services to the public (Kankeu et al., 2016; Kankeu & Ventelou, 2016; Njong & Ngantcha, 2013; Yamb & Bayemi, 2017).

With regards to RQ2, the results revealed organizational change as the main theme and described several measures that hospital managers, policy makers and the government consider in diminishing corrupt business and management practices, including implementing internal and external audit boards, installing anti-corruption bodies, educate and empower the public, and increase employee pay/salary to reduce corruption. managers should engage all stakeholders to solicit their suggestions for improving management processes for enhancing success. As PHS managers, policy makers and the government begin to adopt and implement the resultant stakeholder understandings and measures for diminishing corrupt business and management practices, the likelihood of diminishing it will increase.

Chapter 5

Implications, Recommendations, and Conclusions

Implications

Study implications are discussed per the findings of each research question, including its resultant themes in answer to the problem, purpose, contributions, and implication of the study as supported in the existent scholarship and theory. The key points of the findings are summarized as conclusions.

RQ1: How do stakeholders perceive corrupt business and management practices of bribery in receiving better care at in-patient facilities, unjustified absence and tardiness while being paid, maintaining a "nice" position and promoting and hiring family members to exist in the PHS of Cameroon?

Theme 1: Mismanagement. The findings to the question was that management had failed in its core responsibilities to put in place rules and policies to mitigate corruptive practices in relation to the treatment of patients in triage and leading to prevent patient neglect, measuring staff daily output performance to enhance performance, hold corrupt officials accountable for reducing corruption, provide verbal and financial motivation to staff members to boost morale and employee attitudes towards clients, and hire more staff to reduce exhaustion. According to stakeholder normative principle, management's key responsibilities involves balancing competing interest and giving equal consideration to all stakeholder claims in terms of implementing rules and processes that is fair and transparent to all stakeholders (Donaldson & Preston, 1995; Freeman, 1984).

Consistent with stakeholder theory, Brady and Davies (2014) argued that project failures, including cost overruns and delays within project management settings such as hospitals and information technology depend on how effective project managers can effectively ensure processes and rules for properly identifying key stakeholder competencies are followed to enhance project success. Similarly, Harrison et al.; (2015) affirmed that an agency that manages for its stakeholders ensures its survivability and success. These contentions were affirmed by the findings that rules and processes for treating patients in triage are not properly communicated, outdated, and not followed leading to patient neglect and even death.

The findings implied the need for implementing new and/or revising existing policies and rules for measuring daily staff output performance to enhance quality of service offered to the public. Another implication of the findings is the need for establishing a strong anti-corruption committee that is anchored in the legal system to hold staff members accountable for their actions thus, mitigating impunity and corruption. Consistent with the implication for establishing strong anti-corruption bodies that are centered in the legal system, Kagotho et al.; (2016) revealed that countries in Europe and North America have less corruption than those in Sub Saharan Africa because they have strong anti-corruption bodies such as court system and police with legal authority to investigate and punish corrupt officials thus, preventing its existence.

Another implication of the findings is that managers may be able to attend to the issue of patient neglect in triage by ensuring that its rules and policies are constantly updated and communicated to staff members to increase awareness and reduce neglect. This might be accomplished by increasing the employee response time interval for answering and responding to patient calls for assistance. A foremost implication of the findings is that managers may develop and implement policies to increase transparency in the recruitment and hiring process. Such policies might be design to sanction and penalize officials and/or hiring managers who effectuate employment to family and/or friends without prior publicity of the vacancy. This might be accomplished by ensuring that when job vacancies become available, recruitment should be conducted by a panel of at least five persons, excluding the vote holder with direct supervision of the potential slate of candidate pool.

Theoretically, PHS managers and the Ministry of Public Health (MoPH) will not be able to mitigate corrupt business and management practices until they themselves become aware of the perceived understandings and views of its stakeholders and engage others to the issue of corruption and corruption mitigation. Educational awareness programs and campaigns designed to mitigate corruption and its likelihood of occurring might include management, employee, and public awareness training as to the ills of corruption, including instilling a culture of public service (Chidi, 2013; Mengistu et al., 2013). Chidi (2013) revealed that when citizens are better educated, they are more likely to assess and report corruptive practices thus, reducing its occurrence.

Within the context of the current literature, Tinyami et al.; (2015) had revealed that employees made payments to managers to maintain a "juicy" position and avoid being transferred to rural areas; however, the findings of the current study revealed that employees pay bribes to managers to obtain and maintain their positions because securing and maintaining a job in Cameroon is very difficult due to the high rate of unemployment. As such, the finding of this question was a new revelation and contributed to the existing literature by shedding light on the nature and extent of corruption than can and does occur within the hospital system when managers fail to put in place policies to enhance transparency in the recruitment and hiring process. The findings bore implications for corruption in the hiring process and implied the need for developing legislation and policies that prioritizes transparency in the recruitment and hiring process and for encouraging investment in job creation thus, reducing the likelihood for bribing officials for obtaining and maintaining a job.

Subtheme 1: Motivation. The findings were that management had failed in consistently motivate employees by providing financial and verbal motivation for their hard work. From a normative stakeholder perspective, scholars (Freeman et al., 2007; Tantalo & Priem, 2014) contended that when managers are responsive to stakeholder demands, it enhances stakeholder collaboration and increases agency value thus, enhancing performance. Brady and Davies (2014) affirmed that when project managers provide consistent motivation, including providing financial incentives and recognition, it results to project success, including cost savings due to early project completion. King (2015) contend that agency decisions should consider the interest of all stakeholders by engaging and responding to their demands. These suggestions were supported by the finding that "an employee who is not fully motivated socially and financially will be vulnerable to corruption."

However, the finding that staff/client influence rather than only motivation was a rationale for stakeholder engagement in corruption as there exists some form of motivational incentive in the hospital system though it is small was a new revelation. As such, from a stakeholder theoretical perspective, the findings of the question contributed to stakeholder theory by shedding light on the nature and extent of corruption that occurs within hospital system when managers fail to consistently motivate its employees. The results bore implications of low staff morale and job satisfaction and the need by PHS managers to implement monthly and quarterly financial incentive programs and other reward programs such as service awards, letter of appreciation, and on the spot monetary reward incentives to boost employee morale thus, enhancing employee job satisfaction levels and performance thus, mitigating the likelihood for engaging in corruption.

Within the context of the current literature, the finding that management had failed in consistently provide verbal and financial reward to motivate staff members for exceptional job performance and implied the need for implementing quarterly and monthly employee financial motivational programs when employees exceed performance goals. Consistent with Yamb and Bayemi (2017) corruption within public hospitals in the Littoral Region of Cameroon is due to a lack of motivation and providing verbal and financial motivation might help in enhancing employee job satisfaction, performance, and reducing corruption. Similarly, Agbiboa (2012) argued that providing consistent monetary and financial motivation to civil servants might help in reducing corruption in Nigeria.

Subtheme 2: Low Compensation. The finding was that employees engage corruption and other dubious activities because their salaries are very low as management and the government are not taking steps to increase it. Otherwise, there was no discussion on low compensation perspectives and organizational function with regards to stakeholder perceptions. Thus, the findings may be seen as a contribution (a construct) to stakeholder theory. The findings bore implication for managers and the government for revising its existing compensation plans to ensure its pay levels are in line with those in the private sector thus, mitigating the need for employees to leave work early to attend to another job and engage in dubious activities to augment their salaries.

Consistent with previous research studies, Hope (2014) revealed that corruption in public hospitals in Kenya were due to the low pay of civil servants and suggested the need for the government to increase civil servant pay in order to reduce corruption. Similarly, An and Kweon (2017) showed a significant and positive relationship between pay levels and corruption in developing countries such as Sub Sahara Africa. These arguments were supported by the finding that "because of low salaries/pay, it creates a feeling of "dissatisfaction.""

The findings implied the need for managers and the government (MoPH) to adopt policies for increasing employee pay/salary. This might be accomplished by ensuring that such pay increases are harmonized across the hospital system and are in line with those in the private sector thus, reducing the likelihood for employees to demand, accept bribes, and leave work early in order to work in a second job. Furthermore, such pay increases should be periodically reviewed and adjusted for inflation and align with gross domestic production (GDP) models to ensure its effectiveness thus, preventing and/or mitigating the likelihood of corruption to occur.

Subtheme 3: Staff Shortage. The findings were that there exists an acute shortage of staff given the number of clients served and management has failed to hire more staff to balance staff/client ratio thus, resulting to absenteeism, staff exhaustion, and corruption in bribe for immediate attention by clients and their care givers. Otherwise, there was no argument on staff shortage perspectives and organizational function with regards to stakeholder understanding. Thus, the findings may be seen as a contribution (a construct) to stakeholder theory. The implication of this is that PHS managers cannot attend to the issue of corruption until they are aware of the issues raised by its stakeholders. Launching a hiring program to hire additional workers on a short-term and part-time basis might help in alleviating staff exhaustion thus, enhancing patient care and mitigate corruption.

In previous research, Kankeu et al.; (2016) had revealed that family members and patients make bribe payments to nurses as a condition for accessing and receiving better treatment and care services; however, the findings of the current study that because of acute staff shortage, clients and their carers offer bribes to nurses when they are not asking for it in order to receive special attention from the nurse on duty thus, implying that clients, including their "carers" (family members who care for sick patients while in hospital) are influencing staff members to engage in corruption. As such, the finding was a new revelation and contributed to current literature by shedding light into the nature and extent of corruption than can and does occur in the hospital system because of staff shortage. The findings implied the need to implement policies to ensure that the ratio of staff members to clients is sufficient in accomplishing the desired task thus, mitigating the possibility of clients and their carers to offer bribes to nurses for immediate attention.

Theme 2: High Unemployment. The findings were that employees paid bribes to superiors to secure and maintain a "juicy" position because securing a job is hard due to the high rate of unemployment in Cameroon as those who enter the system try to maintain it. Otherwise, there was no debate on high unemployment perspectives and corruption with regards to stakeholder understanding. Thus, the findings may be seen as a contribution (a construct) to stakeholder theory. The implication of this is for the government, policy makers and managers to develop legislation to spur entrepreneurship by providing investment loans with low interest rates thus, increasing job creation.

In a previous study, Tinyami et al.; (2015) had revealed that doctors and other staff members pay bribes to superiors to avoid being transferred to rural areas and for maintaining a "nice" position; however, the finding of the current study that paying bribes to maintain a "nice" position was because of the high rate of unemployment in Cameroon was a new revelation. As such, the finding contributed to existing literature by uncovering the extent and nature of corruption than can and does occur due in the hospital system due to high unemployment.

The findings bore implication for managers, policy makers, and the government to adopt and implement programs to ensure that when open positions become available, they should be properly advertised in all job boards within the hospital system and the public, including local newspapers, social media sites, and television to inform both internal and external applicants about the job thus, increasing transparency in the hiring process and reducing the likelihood of corruption.

RQ1a. How do stakeholders perceive other corrupt business and management practices that may exist in the PHS of Cameroon?

The findings revealed three other forms of corrupt business and management practices that had not been discussed in the current study and includes the following (a) diversion, (b) extortion, and (c) embezzlement.

Theme 1: Diversion. The findings were that staff members and specifically physicians and health specialists regularly divert patients to private hospitals in which they have a direct financial interest after seeing clients in the office was a new revelation. The findings that health technicians (laboratory technicians, physiotherapists, dental engineers) and some medical specialists, including surgeons, gynecologists, and orthodontists) conduct private practice in the hospital in which they collect money from the client while rendering a service and fail to report and/or record the service(s) rendered, including money paid had not been previously known and can be seen as a contribution for both theory and current literature. Otherwise, there was no discussion on diversion as a form of corruption and organizational function with regards to stakeholder understanding. Thus, the findings may be viewed as a contribution (a construct) to stakeholder theory. The findings bore implication for acute impunity implying the need for implementing policies to ensure that staff guilty of patient deviation, receiving payments without initiating a formal record of the transaction are investigated, punished financially and even judicially thus, mitigating the prospect of its occurrence.

Within the context of the current scholarly literature and the current study, employee perceptions of diversion as a form of corruption has not received much scholarly attention. The findings suggest that employees engage in diversion as a means to augment their low pay/salaries given the monetary motive involved in the practices thus, implying the need for PHS managers to adopt policies design to increase pay/salaries and reduce the chance of employees to engage in such practices. Consistent with the suggestion, Ann and Kweon (2017) revealed a significant relationship between increases in employee pay, levels of corruption and job satisfaction in developing countries such as in Sub Saharan Africa. Similarly, Yamb & Bayemi (2017) have suggested increasing pay levels of public employees within public hospitals in the Littoral province of Cameroon as a measure for reducing corruption.

Theme 2: Extortion. The findings were that staff members, including physicians and nurses abuse their position by extorting money from patients by conditioning type of care provided to level of patronage received. It also revealed that medical specialists such as gynecologists extort money from expectant mothers by charging $266 for a Caesarean Section (C/S) instead of $71 as directed by the government. From a stakeholder theoretical perspective and within the context of this study, stakeholder perceptions of extortion as a form of corruption has not received scholarly attention. As such, the findings might be considered a contribution (a new construct) for stakeholder

127

theory. The findings of this question bore implications for an acute lack of accountability and implying the need for establishing anti-corruption bodies to investigate and hold corrupt officials accountable for their actions. Specifically, such anti-corruption measures might include (a) putting information on notice boards about the wrong doings of the staff, (b) making available the phone numbers of anti-corruption officials to facilitate reporting of corrupt activities by clients and other staff members, and (c) installing cameras in all unit wards and other high corruption service areas.

Current scholarly literature by authors (Kankeu et al., 2016; Yamb & Bayemi, 2017) revealed that hospital staff members illegally keep and sell anti-retroviral drugs such as the Human Immune Virus and Acquired Immune Deficiency Syndrome which are supposed to be free to patients supported the findings that physicians operate a mini pharmacy in their office for sale to clients and were to be expected given the corruption in the hospital system. However, the finding that medical specialists such as gynecologists extort money from expectant mothers by charging $266 for a C/S instead of $71 as stipulated by the government was a new revelation and thus, can be viewed as a contribution for existing scholarship.

The finding implied the need for PHS managers and the government for designing and implementing educational programs design to educate and empower the public and public employees about the ills of corruption and the right of citizens when visiting and receiving health care related services within in-patient and out-patient hospital facilities. Such educational programs and curriculum should instill a culture of service excellence in young people and the ills of corruption and by posting in hospital notice boards official costs for medical procedures, including lab fees, C/S procedures, and medications.

Consistent with this argument, Chidi (2014) revealed that empowering individuals through educational programs enable them to have an awareness about corruption and interest in ensuring that best business practices are strictly enforced thus, reducing corruption. Walton and Peiffer (2017) revealed that levels of education positively influenced public assessment of corrupt practices in public institutions as educated individuals are more likely to report corrupt activities to authorities than less educated ones thus, reducing its occurrence. When employees (nurses, nurse managers, physicians) are educated and informed they are more likely to monitor and report corrupt practices to appropriate management and government officials thus, diminishing its likelihood of occurring (Fortunato & Panizza, 2015; Walton & Peiffer, 2017).

Theme 3: Embezzlement. The findings were that top-level hospital officials embezzle funds appropriated by the government for infrastructure development and procurement of hospital equipment as patients in need of specialized services are forced to seek medical care out of their area of residence in neighboring towns and out of Cameroon. According to stakeholder normative principle, management's core actions and responsibilities should be on the agency and its stakeholders and from the stakeholders to the agency for enhancing value creation and agency success (Donaldson & Preston, 1995; Freeman, 1984; Tantalo & Priem, 2014). Tantalo and Priem (2014) observed that when management's actions affect another stakeholder, it prevents effective stakeholder collaboration and reduces value creation for all stakeholders.

The discussion was affirmed by the finding that because of embezzlement by top managers patients requiring specialized services have to seek care out of their area of residence in neighboring towns and at times out of Cameroon and resulting to extra monetary costs. Theoretically, the findings contributed to stakeholder theory by enhancing understanding of the nature

129

and extend of embezzlement and what can and does occur when public officials embezzle public funds. The findings implied the need for managers in establishing an audit board (internal and external) to ensure checks and balances in how hospital projects are managed. Ayuso et al.; (2014) revealed that firms with independent audit boards, including internal and external organs are more likely to increase the level of confidence among stakeholders than those that do not and leading to a high degree of trust among investors. At a general level, the findings imply that organizations with higher activities of quality management practices such as audit boards and complying with financial disclosure requirements are more likely to be more responsible to all its stakeholders.

Within the context of current scholarly literature, the findings that top managers embezzle hospital funds meant for infrastructure improvements were consistent with the study by Agbiboa (2012) that revealed management level corruption in the form of embezzlement in Nigeria. Similarly, Njong and Ngantcha (2013) revealed management level corruption within the health care delivery chain in Cameroon where hospital officials abuse funds meant for buying supplies and equipment. Equally, Osifo (2014) affirmed corruption by top managers within public hospitals in Nigeria and Cameroon so that the findings that top managers within the PHS embezzle funds were expected. The findings contributed to current literature by shedding light on the nature and extend of embezzlement within the hospital system.

The findings bore implication of a severe corruption thus, implying the need for PHS managers and the government to create (V.I.P) health services facilities in all big public hospitals in cities and/or towns with populations of more than 500,000 inhabitants to reduce cost on receiving care. This might be achieved by ensuring that the service facilities have all the requisite care services, including better trained personnel and

130

equipment thus, helping to reduce medical related costs, including travel and lodging in seeking better care in other cities and/or towns.

RQ2. How do stakeholders perceive ways to diminish and improve the business and management practices that exist in the PHS of Cameroon?

Stakeholder responses to this question resulted in the identification of one theme organizational change. The findings yielded an overarching theme, organizational change (empowerment, accountability, motivation, and increase compensation) as measures for diminishing corruption.

Theme 1: Organizational Change. The finding was that in order to mitigate corruptive business and management practices, hospital managers and the MoPH should adopt policies, rules, and regulations, including strengthening anti-corruption bodies, installing an internal and external audit board, streamline decision-making processes to engage key stakeholders, empower denizens, and increase compensation. According to stakeholder strategic management practices for success, stakeholder theorists Gupta & Sharma (2014) contend that when good governance practices consisting a combination of policies, rules, laws on ways to manage an agency such as, stakeholder engagement, proper internal audit controls requirements, and an independent management board, it led to improved agency performance and success of Indian and South Korean firms.

In line with this argument, Ayuso et al.; (2014) revealed a significant and positive relationship between a firm's internal audit board processes, including its financial disclosure records and increase in level of confidence among stakeholders leading to a high degree of trust among investors. This discussion was

131

supported by the findings that PHS managers should implement internal and external audit boards to increase financial transparency to mitigate corruption. Consistent with the findings that PHS managers should decentralize management processes to include and engage key stakeholders in the decision-making process, Brady and Davies (2014) and Eskerod et al.; (2015) argued that when stakeholders are not properly engaged in agency decision-making processes, the potential for project failure increases. Similarly, King (2015) contend that agency decisions should consider the interest of all stakeholders by engaging and soliciting their opinions.

Other stakeholder theorists (Pandi-Perumal et al., 2015; Starks et al., 2015) have suggested stakeholder engagement as a management practice that seek to involve stakeholders in a positive manner in all aspects involving organizational actions to enhance success. Starks et al.; (2015), for example, revealed that when key stakeholders were involved in the decision-making process of creating treatment programs for depression within Indian reservations in the state of Alaska, it resulted in the creation of early detection programs for diagnosing depression and reduction in depression among young adults. These arguments were in line with the findings that managers should streamline the decision-making process to include employees. However, the revelation that management and the government should create V.I.P health facilities in towns with populations of more than 500,000 inhabitants to improve quality of care, reduce costs to clients and prevent corruption in bribes in order to receive better care service and hire more staff to increase patient/staff ratio to reduce patient queue and corruption were new. As such, the revelations contributed to stakeholder theory by enhancing understanding of measures that managers might implement to enhance agency performance and long-term success.

In current scholarly literature, Agbiboa (2012) suggested the need for government and civil service managers to create and strengthen anti-corruption bodies as a measure for reducing widespread corruption in the Nigerian public sector. Similarly, Hope (2014) affirmed the creation of strong anti-corruption bodies that are anchored in sound legal systems for reducing corruption within Kenyan public hospital. However, the findings also revealed that PHS managers in order to mitigate corruption, managers should decentralize the management of hospital functions and involve heads of units and chief of services who should be qualified personnel within their respective departments in the decision-making process to reduce corruption.

As such, the finding contributed to current literature as to how managers might engage employees to better manage agency processes. The findings bore implication of a lack of good governance practices thus, implying the need for implementing policies for streamlining the decision-making process (King, 2015). This can be achieved by ensuring that peripheral administrators (ward charges, unit heads and key employees) are involved and consulted in the early decision-making processes. This might include joint discussions in the early adoption and implementation of patient centric approaches in enhancing care services such as increasing the response time of nurses in responding to patients after receiving a call for assistance. According to Starks et al. (2015) when key stakeholders are involved in the decision-making process of creating treatment programs for depression within Indian reservations in the state of Alaska, it led to the creation of early detection programs for diagnosing depression that reduced depression among young adults.

Sub theme 1: Empowerment. The findings were that PHS managers, policy makers, and the government should design and adopt policies to empower unit heads and ward charges to take disciplinary actions on corruption within their departments to reduce corruption and educative programs within school systems design to sensitize the public within about the ills of corruption, including their rights while receiving care services in health facilities. From a stakeholder theoretical and within the context of this study, stakeholder perceptions of empowerment as a measure for reducing corruption has not received scholarly attention thus, the findings contributed to stakeholder theory.

Within the context of the current literature, the findings were consistent with Walton and Peiffer's (2017) study that revealed education base corruptive programs can positively influence the public's assessment of corrupt practices in public institutions as educated individuals are more likely to report corrupt activities to authorities than less educated ones, thus diminishing its likelihood of occurring. Similarly, Fortunato and Panizza (2015) revealed a significant relationship between levels of education and good governance practices. Chidi (2014) contended that education-based corruption programs enable individuals to have an awareness and interest in ensuring that best business practices, including merit-based selection, hiring and promotion policies are strictly enforced thus, leading to less corruption. Otherwise, there was no discussion on perceived empowerment as a measure for diminishing corruptive business and management practices.

The finding implied the need for implementing early education awareness programs in schools to teach citizens from an early age about the ills of corruption and empower them about their rights to services while in hospital facilities and empowering peripheral administrators, including unit heads and ward charges by giving them disciplinary authority to address lateness, absenteeism, and other malign behaviors that affect work output to reduce corruption. The findings also imply that crafting educational programs specifically design for children and young adults from K-12 might help in instilling a culture of integrity about public service thus, empowering them to better assess and report corruption.

Another implication of the finding is the need for managers working with the Ministry of Education to develop anti-corruption base educational programs design to impart a culture of anti-corruption awareness among the population thus, dissuading citizens from engaging in corrupt activities and reducing its likelihood of occurring (Chidi, 2014; Walton & Peiffer, 2017). Another implication of the finding is that managers might be able to extend disciplinary authority to peripheral managers to who work at the unit level to better assess and make decisions on corrupt activities such as absenteeism and sale of drugs thus, reducing the prospect of such practices from occurring.

Sub theme 2: Accountability. The findings were that management and the government should implement a system of accountability, including internal and external audit board control and strong anti-corruption committees in all hospital units and departments with authority to hold corrupt officials accountable for their actions. From a stakeholder theoretical perspective, when accountability measures, including independent audit board are instituted, it leads to greater transparency and enhanced stakeholder confidence. Consistent with stakeholder theory, Ayuso et al.; (2014) revealed a significant and positive relationship between a firm's audit board processes, including its financial disclosure records and increase in the level of confidence among stakeholders and leading to a high degree of trust.

Similarly, Chan et al.; (2014) affirmed that agencies that consistently apply good governance practices, including independent audit boards and proper financial disclosure information as a management strategy are more likely to enhance their performance and value creation for its stakeholders than those that do not. These contentions were in line with the finding that in order to reduce corruption, managers would need to setup strong audit control system both internally and externally to ensure checks and balances between the bodies. Theoretically, PHS managers and the MoPH cannot mitigate corruption unless they themselves aware of the views of their stakeholders. Implementing internal and external audit boards to ensure greater accountability of finances and ensuring projects are properly procured and executed might reduce corruption and enhance confidence among all stakeholders.

Within the context of the current literature and as with the theme organizational change, the findings that managers should implement anti-corruption committees in all units to investigate and punish corrupt practices supported the findings of Agbiboa (2012) in which he suggested the need for government and civil service managers to create and strengthen anti-corruption bodies as a measure for reducing widespread corruption in Nigerian public sector. Hope (2014) affirmed the creation of strong anti-corruption bodies that are anchored in sound legal systems for reducing corruption within Kenyan public hospital. However, the findings of specific anti-corruption measures design to diminish corruption namely: (a) putting information on notice boards concerning the wrong doings of the staff, (b) making available the phone numbers of anti-corruption officials to facilitate reporting of corrupt activities by clients and other staff members, and (c) installing cameras in all unit wards and other high corruption service areas were new revelations. As such, the findings contributed to current literature by enhancing understanding as to the policies that managers and the government might consider for reducing corruption. The implications of this is that in order to hold officials and employees' accountable, managers and the government might consider installing strong anti-corruption bodies to investigate and severely punish those guilty of engaging in corrupt activities.

This might be done by installing cameras in all hospital units to monitor and punish corruption.

Consistent with current literature, Agbiboa (2012) suggested the need for the Nigerian government and civil service managers to create and strengthen anti-corruption bodies to investigate and punish corrupt officials as a measure for reducing widespread corruption in the public sector. Hope (2014) affirmed the creation of strong anti-corruption bodies that are anchored in sound legal systems as a way for reducing corruption within Kenyan public hospitals. The findings implied the need for managers for instituting quality management practices such as independent audit boards and anti-corruption panels for enhancing transparency thus, reducing corruption (Gupta & Sharma, 2014).

Sub theme 3: Motivation. The findings were that managers should adopt and implement policies that seek to consistently provide financial and verbal motivation, including personal recognition to staff members when they do an excellent job to boost morale and increase worker attitudes and behaviors towards clients and the agency. Stakeholder management responsibilities involve balancing competing interests in terms of adopting and implementing policies, including providing financial incentives and recognition for exceptional service in a way that creates value for all stakeholders and ensures the survival of the agency (Donaldson & Preston, 1995; Freeman, 1984).

Within stakeholder project management settings such as engineering and hospitals that have several departments, including unit and department heads, Brady and Davies (2014) revealed that when project managers implemented employee motivation programs, including providing financial incentives, it resulted to increased job satisfaction rates and led to early project completion rates and cost savings. These arguments were consistent with the finding that managers should consistently provide verbal and monetary motivation. The findings bore implication for an acute lack of employee job satisfaction and implying the need for designing policies and programs for providing quarterly monetary incentives and recognition to employees for exceeding output performance.

Consistent with current scholarly scholarship, Yamb and Bayemi (2017) revealed that corruption within public hospitals in Douala Cameroon was a result of lack of staff motivation by management and suggested that in order to reduce corruption, hospital managers and the government of Cameroon should consider providing financial incentives for enhancing job satisfaction and reducing corruption. Likewise, Agbiboa (2012) suggested that providing motivational incentives may help in reducing public corruption in Nigeria. Similarly, Kagotho et al.; (2016) suggested that providing financial motivation may increase public sector worker morale in Kenya and reduce corruption. These contentions are in line with the finding that managers should consistently motivate staffs for their efforts and specifically anti-corruption employees to spur them to do their jobs with due diligence."

The findings implied an acute lack of employee motivation with implications for corruption and organizational success thus, implying that in order to reduce corruption, managers should implement policies that ensure they are consistently providing verbal and financial motivation to employees. This might include daily verbal appreciation and service excellence recognition (medals, letters, notes and gifts) to boost employee morale thus improving employee attitudes towards clients and the agency. Financial rewards might include providing incentives per each department and unit (Agbiboa, 2012; Hope, 2014; Yamb & Bayemi, 2017).

Sub theme 4: Increase Compensation. The findings were that management and the government should increase employee pay/salary to boost morale and reduce the need for employees to engage in corrupt activities. Within the context of stakeholder theory and this study, the theme, increase compensation as a measure for mitigating corruption has not received scholarly attention. As such, the findings may be viewed as a new construct (contribution) for stakeholder theory.

Within the context of the current literature, the findings that management should increase employee salaries/pay is consistent with Yamb and Bayemi's (2017) study in which they suggested in order to reduce corruption within public hospitals in the Littoral Region of Cameroon, the government should increase civil servant salaries/pay. Similarly, Kagotho et al.; (2016) suggested that to reduce public sector corruption in Kenya, the government should increase public employee pay. An and Kweon (2017) also revealed a significant relationship between increases in public employee pay and low-levels of corruption especially in developing countries such as Sub Sahara Africa like Cameroon. A foremost implication of the findings is that increasing employees pay/salary may be helpful in mitigating corruption as it might help in boosting employee morale and level of job satisfaction thus, their attitudes towards clients and the agency (An & Kweon, 2017; Yamb & Bayemi, 2017). This might be accomplished by ensuring that such pay/salary increases are harmonized across the public sector and taking into consideration market prices and adjusted with inflation.

Finally, having used the stakeholder theoretical framework to understand and explain the views of PHS stakeholders, this study contributed to the tenants of the theory. The thrust of stakeholder theory is that organizational success is dependent upon the ability of managers to build effective relationships while upholding the interest of all its stakeholders (Freeman, 1984; Freeman, 2011; Tantalo & Priem, 2013). Freeman (1984; 2011) and Tantalo and Priem (2013) contended that in order to enhance organizational success and long-term firm survival, managers must build and maintain effective relationships, while

139

balancing the interests of the firm with those of all its stakeholders (Freeman & Phillips, 2002). From a PHS management perspective, it implies that in order to diminish corruption in the hospital system, PHS managers would need to be aware of stakeholder perceived interest in corruption, rationale for corruption and the measures for diminishing it (Freeman, 1984; Freeman & Phillips, 2002). As managers, the government, and policy makers begin to acquaint themselves and implement the resultant measures for diminishing corruption, the likelihood for its occurrence might reduce.

Recommendations for Practical Application

The findings of the research questions resulted in the identification of nine measures that might help for diminishing corruption. The measures that are recommended for practical application are discussed below.

As a way for improving the quality of care services provided to the public, reducing travel related costs in seeking services, and diminish corruption in the demands for bribes in receiving better care services at the hospital system, a need was revealed for creating (V.I.P) health service facilities that are fully staffed with better trained personnel and equipment in all cities and/or towns with a population of more than 500,000 inhabitants (Kankeu et al., 2016; Yamb & Bayemi, 2017). Such V.I.P health facilities would be able to provide the requisite care services needed by clients within their communities thus, diminishing corruption in bribes by employees in order to provide better care to clients (Kankeu et al., 2016). Creating V.I.P care facilities in all major towns might be helpful in reducing travel related costs such as transportation that are borne by individuals in seeking specialized services in other cities and out of Cameroon thus, increasing the likelihood of clients to seek preventative care (Kankeu et al., 2016; Njong & Ngantcha, 2013).

140

As another measure for enhancing employee job attitudes and behavior towards clients and diminish the likelihood for engaging in corrupt activities, a need to increase employee pay/salary was reveled in the current study (Agbiboa, 2012; Yamb & Bayemi, 2017). Managers need to ensure that salary/pay increases are in-line with those in the private sector and harmonize across the hospital system to ensure pay equity and fairness (Yamb & Bayemi, 2017). Salary/pay increases might help in boosting staff morale and thus their attitudes and behaviors towards to clients and reduce the likelihood to engage in corrupt activities (An & Kweon, 2017; Hope, 2014; Kagotho et al., 2016).

As a method for enhancing organizational and staff efficiency, the need for implementing daily staff output performance measurement was revealed in the current study (Kagotho et al., 2016; Yamb & Bayemi, 2017). Staff daily output performance measurements would help managers in ensuring employees are meeting agency prescribed performance goals and in identifying areas of weaknesses that may require additional training thus, allowing the development and design of extra training programs design to improve efficiency and overall agency performance and long-term success (Mengistu et al., 2013; Tantalo & Priem, 2015).

As a way of reducing staff exhaustion that results from acute staff shortage and the corruption in staff/client influence (where care givers offer bribes to nurses to receive special attention due to staff shortage), a need for hiring more qualified staff was revealed in the current study. Additional staff members would help to reduce staff exhaustion by making equal the ratio of nurses to patients thus, preventing the need for clients to offer bribes to nurses for receiving special and/or immediate attention (Fongwa, 2002; Kankeu et al., 2017).

As a means for demonstrating to employees that their hard work is valued and appreciated by managers, it was identified in the current study for managers to consistently motivate employees by providing financial reward and verbal recognition. Financial reward payments might include quarterly and semi-annual cash bonuses for meeting or exceeding measurable performance goals (Hope, 2014; Yamb & Bayemi, 2017). Additional recognition awards might include designing service excellence recognition programs and policies for rewarding longevity in service and might include medals and personal letters from managers to employees. Providing consistent verbal and financial rewards will help motivate and increase job satisfaction levels among employees thus, enhancing the overall job performance (Agbiboa, 2012; Kagotho et al., 2016).

As a measure for improving managerial decision-making and ensuring agency processes, including procedures and policies for treating patients in the triage are constantly updated and properly community to staff, a need for decentralizing managerial decision-making processes to include peripheral administrators, including unit heads, department managers, and employees in the decision-making process was revealed in the current study (Ayuso et al., 2014; Starks et al., 2015). Managers should engage and/or include unit heads, department managers, and lead staff members in organizational discussions in developing, designing, and implementing patient centric approaches for treating patients in triage. Including stakeholders in the decision-making process might lead to new and improved methods for increasing the response time in attending to and treating patients in triage thus, reducing patient neglect and even death (Ayuso et al., 2014; Kankeu et al., 2016; Starks et al., 2015).

In order to diminish corruption in diversion, where some doctors keep a small pharmacy in their offices for sale to patients, refer patients to private clinics for consultations after seeing them in the hospital, and in extortion, where medical professionals such as Gynecologists charged expectant mothers $266 for C/S services instead of $71 as mandated by the government, the need for creating strong anti-corrupt committees in all units and departments that are anchored in the legal system to investigate and severely penalize corrupt officials was revealed in the current study (Agbiboa, 2012; Kagotho et al., 2016). Specifically, to ensure the effectiveness of the anti-corruption bodies, managers should consider the following measures: (a) putting information on notice boards about the wrong doings of the staff, (b) making available the phone numbers of anti-corruption officials to facilitate reporting of corrupt activities by clients and other staff members, (c) installing cameras in unit wards and other high corruption service areas, and (d) setting up disciplinary councils in each department to investigate corrupt activities.

As a means for empowering citizens to better assess and report corruption and be inform about their rights when visiting hospital facilities, the need for creating education-based programs in schools was identified in the current study (Chidi, 2013). Educational programs might be design to sensitize the public about the ills of corruption on national development. Education-based anti-corruption programs might reduce corruption by developing a culture of public service among individuals by giving them the tools to better assess and report corrupt activities thus, reducing its likelihood of occurring (Mengistu et al., 2013; Walton & Peiffer, 2017).

Finally, as a way of reducing corruption in collected fees, embezzlement of appropriated funds for infrastructure development, and enhance transparency in undocumented receipts paid, the need for creating accounting standards by creating an internal and external audit board was identified in the current study (Osifo, 2014; Sabella et al., 2014). Audit boards should have checks and balances to ensure transparency and its independence. Audit board controls might help in reducing corruption in embezzlement, corruption in collected fees, and enhance transparency among its stakeholders thus, increasing

143

the public's confidence in the hospital system and its overall mission of improving the well-being of the public (Sabella et al., 2014; Tantalo & Priem, 2015).

Recommendations for Future Research

Findings of the current study resulted in the identification of nine specific measures design to diminish corruption; however, they are yet to be adopted and/or implemented to ascertain its effectiveness in mitigating corruption. As such, they can be seen as a potential limitation of the study requiring additional research.

As a means for reducing corruption in diversion, where some doctors keep a small pharmacy in their offices for sale to patients, refer patients to private clinics for consultations after seeing them in the hospital, and in extortion in extortion, where medical professionals such as Gynecologists charged expectant mothers for $266 C/S services instead of $71 as mandated by the government, a need for creating strong anti-corruption bodies that are legally grounded to investigate and punish corrupt officials and reduce corruption was identified in the current study (Hope, 2014; Kagotho et al., 2016; Nguemegne, 2011; Osifo, 2014). Strong anti-corruption bodies that are legally grounded are vital for reducing corruption in (Kagotho et al., 2016; Nguemegne, 2011). However, research on the requirements for setting up anti-corrupt bodies that are legally anchored in the legal system to reduce corruption is lacking in the existing literature. Additional research is recommended for investigating the requirements for setting up such anti-corruption bodies. Such research might qualitatively be design to include other public hospitals facing similar issues with corruption and using research questions that asks stakeholder perceptions of ways in designing and implementing such bodies (Kagotho et al., 2016; Nguemegne, 2011).

144

As a means for reducing corruption in collected fees, embezzlement of appropriated funds for infrastructure development, and enhance transparency in undocumented receipts paid, the need for creating an internal and external audit board to provide checks and balances and enhance stakeholder confidence in the hospital system was identified in the current study (Osifo, 2014; Sabella et al., 2014). However, quality management practices in audit board controls are lacking within the hospital system as revealed in the current study's findings. Thus, additional research is recommended to investigate how the audit boards might be design to achieve the desired outcome. Such research might qualitatively be design to include more specific open-ended research questions that asks stakeholder working in other similar hospitals and having corruption the perceptions of how the design and implementation of the audit board in terms of its specific policies, rules, procedures, board composition, and independence might affect its effectiveness.

Conclusions

The problem addressed in this qualitative multiple case study was the corrupt business and management practices that continue to lead to increased monetary cost to individuals and delays in seeking preventative care services within the hospital system (Kankeu et al., 2016; Osifo, 2014; Njong & Ngantcha, 2013; Yamb & Bayemi, 2017). The purpose of the study was to provide further understanding of how to diminish corrupt business and management practices that continue to lead to increased monetary cost to individuals and delays in seeking preventative care within the PHS of Cameroon. Semi-structured, open-ended interviews were conducted with nine participants (three nurse managers, three nurses and three physicians) at a regional hospital in the Northwest region of Cameroon (Yin, 2009). Stakeholder theoretical framework is

145

used for understanding and explaining the behaviors and perceptions of hospital employees within the context of organizational governance (Freeman, 1984; Harrison et al., 2015; Hasnas, 2013; Tantalo & Priem, 2014). Specifically, stakeholder theory was used

Thematic analysis of the data resulted in the identification of several themes and subthemes thus, revealing new forms of corruptions, including its nature and extent not previously discussed in previous literature and theory. Within the context of organization function and corruption, the theme high unemployment uncovered that while in previous study Tinyami et al. (2015) had revealed that employees made payments to managers to maintain a "juicy" position and avoid being transferred to rural areas, the current study revealed that employees pay bribes to managers to obtain and maintain their positions because securing and maintaining a job in Cameroon is very difficult due to the high rate of unemployment.

The findings of the study also revealed that although a lack of motivation in the form of verbal and financial reward was a rationale for stakeholder engagement in corruption, it was revealed that a lack of motivation was not the only reason for engaging in corruption as there exists some form of financial incentives in the hospital system, though it was little. In previous studies, researchers (Kankeu et al., 2016; Yamb & Bayemi, 2017) had revealed nurses demand bribes from patients to receive better care; however, the findings revealed that at times clients and their families offer bribes to nurses to receive special attention thus, suggesting that corruption in bribes was due to client influence and not staff thus, contributing to current literature by enhancing understanding of the nature and extent of corruption and can and does occur when managers fail to sufficiently motivate employees (Hope, 2014; Yamb & Bayemi, 2017).

146

Within the context of stakeholder theory and specifically organizational function, the findings contributed to stakeholder theory by revealing two other forms of corruption namely: diversion and extortion. Corruption in diversion and extortion further revealed the nature and extent of the practices where staff members and specifically physicians and health specialists regularly divert patients to private hospitals in which they have a direct financial interest after seeing clients in their office and charging expectant mothers $266 instead of $ 71 for a C/S as mandated by the government. The study findings also resulted in nine specific measures that managers, policy makers and the government might implement design to diminish corruption and used as Recommendations for Practical Application.

Stakeholders perceived the need for empowering citizens to reduce corruption by developing education-based programs to teach them about the ills of corruption, thus allowing them to better assess and report corruption and reducing its likelihood of occurring (Chidi, 2013; Walton & Peiffer, 2017). Additionally, the findings revealed that to enhance managerial effectiveness, managers should engage stakeholders in the decision-making process to help in early discussions in designing patient centric approaches to improving quality of care services provided to the public (Noland & Phillips, 2010; Starks et al., 2015).

Finally, as a way of reducing corruption in collected fees, embezzlement of appropriated funds for infrastructure development, and enhance transparency, the need for creating an internal and external audit board with checks and balances was identified in the study (Osifo, 2014; Sabella et al., 2014). However, quality management practices in audit board controls are lacking within the hospital system. Thus, additional qualitative research is recommended to investigate how such audit boards might be design in terms of its composition, rules, and policies to be effective.

References

Afolayan, A. (2012). Postcolonialism and the two publics' in Nigeria: Rethinking the idea of the skeptical public. *Journal of African Studies*, 9, 44-68. Retrieved from http://dx.doi.org/10.4314/og.v9i1.2

Agbiboa, D. (2012). Between corruption and development: The political economy of state robbery in Nigeria. *Journal of Business Ethics*, *108*(3), 325-345. doi:10.1007/s10551-011-1093-5

Angeles, L., & Neanidis, K. C. (2015). The persistent effect of colonialism on corruption. *Economica*, *82*(326), 319-349. doi: 10.1111/ecca.12123

An, W., & Kweon, Y. (2017). Do higher government wages induce less corruption? Cross-country panel evidence. *Journal of Policy Modeling*, doi:10.1016/j.jpolmod.2017.03.001

Awasum, H. M. (1992). Health and nursing services in Cameroon: Challenges and demands for nurses in leadership positions. *Nursing Administration Quarterly*, 16(2), 8-13. Retrieved from https://www.ncbi.nlm.nih.gov/pubmed/1738498

Abobakr, M. G. (2017). Corporate governance and banks performance: Evidence from Egypt. *Asian Economic and Financial Review*, 7(12), 1326 1343. http://www.aessweb.com/download.php?id=3954

Aguilera, R. V., & Crespi-Cladera, R. (2016). Global corporate governance: On the relevance of firms' ownership structure. *Journal of World Business*, *51*(The World of Global Business 1965-2015), 50-57. doi:10.1016/j.jwb.2015.10.003

Ansoff, I. (1965). *Corporate Strategy:* An analytic approach for business policy for growth and expansion. McGraw-Hill

Asongu, S. A. (2013). Fighting corruption in Africa: do existing corruption-control levels matter? *International Journal of Development Issues, 12*(1), 36-52. doi.org/10.1108/14468951311322109

Ayuso, S., Rodríguez, M. A., García-Castro, R., & Ariño, M. A. (2014). Maximizing stakeholders' interests: An empirical analysis of the stakeholder approach to corporate governance. *Business & society, 53*(3), 414-439. doi/abs/10.1177/0007650311433122

Babnik, K., Breznik, K., Dermol, V., & Širca, N. T. (2014). The mission statement: organizational culture perspective. *Industrial Management & Data Systems, 114*(4), 612 627. doi:10.1108/IMDS-10-2013-0455

Baker, C. (2015). Multilingual literature and official bilingualism in Cameroon: Francis Nyamnjoh's A Nose for Money (2006) and Patrice Nganang's Temps de chien (2001). *International Journal of Francophone Studies, 18*(1), 59-75. doi: https://doi.org/10.1386/ijfs.18.1.59_1

Barnard, C. (1938). *The function of the executive.* Cambridge, MA: Harvard University Press

Birney, M. (2014). Decentralization and veiled corruption under China's "Rule of Mandates." *World Development, 53*55-67. doi:10.1016/j.worlddev.2013.01.006

Bear, S., Rahman, N., & Post, C. (2010). The impact of board diversity and gender composition on corporate social responsibility and firm reputation. Journal of Business Ethics, 97(2), 207–221. doi:10.1007/s10551-010-0505-2

Beschorner, T. (2014). Creating shared value: The one-trick pony approach. *Business Ethics Journal Review, 1*(17), 106-112. http://doi.org.10.12747.bejrl2013.01.17

Berle, A. A., Means, G. (1932). *The Modern Corporation and Private Property.* New York, NY: Transaction Publishers

Beeri, I., & Navot, D. (2013). Local political corruption: Potential structural malfunctions at the central–local, local–

local and intra-local levels. *Public Management Review, 15*(5), 712. doi:10.1080/14719037.2012.707682

Brady, T., & Davies, A. (2014). Managing structural and dynamic complexity: A tale of two projects. *Project Management Journal, 45*(4), 21–38. doi:10.1002/pmj.21434

Braun, V., & Clarke, V. (2006). Using thematic analysis in psychology. *Qualitative research in psychology, 3*(2), 77-101. doi:10.1191/1478088706qp063oa

Brown, J., & Forster, W. (2013). CSR and stakeholder theory: A tale of Adam Smith. *Journal of Business Ethics, 112*(2), 301-312. doi:10.1007/s10551-012-1251-4

Bundy, J., Shropshire, C., & Bucholtz, A. K. (2013). Strategic cognition and issue salience: Toward an explanation of firm responsiveness to stakeholder concerns. *Academy of Management Review,* 38(3), 352–376.

Burkitt, I. (2013). Self and others in the field of perception: The role of micro-dialogue, feeling, and emotion in perception. *Journal of Theoretical and Philosophical Psychology, 33*(4), 267-279. doi:10.1037/a0030255

Carlon, D. M., & Downs, A. (2014). Stakeholder valuing: A process for identifying the interrelationships between firm and stakeholder attributes. *Administrative Sciences 4*(2), 137–154. http://dx.doi.org/10.3390/admsci4020137

Clarke, V., & Braun, V. (2017). Thematic analysis. *Journal of Positive Psychology, 12*(3), 297. doi:10.1080/17439760.2016.1262613

Cording, M., Harrison, J.S., Hoskisson, R.E. and Jonsen, K. (2014). Walking the talk: A multi-stakeholder exploration of organizational authenticity, employee productivity and post-merger performance. *Academy of Management Perspectives,* 28 (1), 38-56. doi:10.5465/amp.2013.0002

Christensen, J., Kent, P., Routledge, J., & Stewart, J. (2015). Do corporate governance recommendations improve the performance and accountability of small listed companies? *Accounting & Finance*, *55*(1), 133-164. doi:10.1111/acfi.12055

Clinton, M. E., & Guest, D. E. (2014). Psychological contract breach and voluntary turnover: Testing a multiple mediation model. *Journal of Occupational and Organizational Psychology*, *87*(1), 200-207. doi:10.1111/joop.12033

Darley, W. K. (2003). Public policy challenges and implications of the Internet and the emerging e-commerce for sub-Saharan Africa: A business perspective. *Information Technology for Development*, *10*(1), 1. doi.10.1002/itdj.1590100102

Donaldson, T., & Preston, L. E. (1995). The stakeholder theory of the corporation: Concepts, evidence and applications. *Academy of Management Review*, *20*(1), 65-91. doi:10.5465/AMR.1995.9503271992

Donchev, D., & Ujhelyi, G. (2014). What do corruption indices measure? *Economics & Politics*, *26*(2), 309-331. doi:10.1111/ecpo.12037

Dong, B., & Torgler, B. (2013). Causes of corruption: Evidence from China. *China Economic Review*, *26*152-169. doi:10.1016/j.chieco.2012.09.005

Djouma, F. N., Ateudjieu, J., Ram, M., Debes, A. K., & Sack, D. A. (2016). Factors associated with fatal outcomes following cholera-like syndrome in Far North Region of Cameroon: A community-based survey. *The American Journal of Tropical Medicine and Hygiene*, *95*(6), 1287-1291.doi: 10.4269/ajtmh.16-0300

Eskerod, P., Huemann, M., & Savage, G. (2015). Project stakeholder management—Past and present. *Project Management Journal*, *46*(6), 6-14. doi:10.1002/pmj.21555

Fongwa, M. (2002). International health care perspectives: the Cameroon example. *Journal of Transcultural Nursing*, *13*(4), 325-330. Retrieved from http://journals.sagepub.com.proxy1.ncu.edu/doi/pdf/10.1177/104365902236708

Fortunato, P., & Panizza, U. (2015). Democracy, education and the quality of government. *Journal of Economic Growth*, *20*(4), 333-363. doi: 10.1007/s10887-015-9120-5

Forson, J., Baah-Ennumh, T., Buracom, P., Chen, G., & Zhen, P. (2016). Causes of corruption: Evidence from sub-Saharan Africa. *South African Journal of Economic and Management Sciences, 19*(4), 562-578. doi:http://dx.doi.org/10.4102/sajems.v19i4.1530

Freeman, R. E. (1984). *Strategic management*: A stakeholder approach. Marshfield, MA: Pitman Books.

Freeman, R. E. (1994). The politics of stakeholder theory. *Business Ethics Quarterly,* 4 (4), 409- 421.doi: 10.2307/3857340

Freeman, H. (1999). Divergent stakeholder theory. *Academy of Management Review, 24*(2), 233-236. doi:10.5465/AMR.1999.1893932

Freeman, R. E. & Phillips, R.A. (2002). Stakeholder theory: A libertarian defense. *Business Ethics Quarterly, 12(3)* 331-349. doi: 10.2139/ssrn.263514

Freeman, R. E. (2011). Managing for stakeholders: Trade-offs or value creation. *Journal of Business Ethics, 96*(1), 7–9. http://dx.doi.org/10.1007/s10551-011-0935-5

Freeman, R. E., Harrison, J. S., Wicks, A. C., Parmar, B. L., & De Colle, S. (2013). *Stakeholder theory: The state of the art.* New York, NY: Cambridge. (Original work published 2010)

Friedman, A.L. and Miles, S. (2006). *"Stakeholders: Theory and Practice."* Oxford, U.K: Oxford University Press.

Fry, L. J. (2016). The search for a culture of bribery in Cameroon. *World Journal of Social Science Research, 3*(2), 185.doi.org/10.22158/wjssr.v3n2p185

Glaeser, E. L. & Shleifer, A. (2002). Legal origins. *Quarterly Journal of Economics,* 117(4):1193-1229. Retrieved from https://scholar.harvard.edu/shleifer/publications/legal origins

Gonin, M. (2015). Adam Smith's contribution to business ethics, then and now. *Journal of Business Ethics*, *129*(1), 221-236. doi:10.1007/s10551-014-2153-4

Hajizadeh, M., Sia, D., Heymann, S. J., & Nandi, A. (2014). Socioeconomic inequalities in HIV/AIDS prevalence in sub-Saharan African countries: evidence from the demographic health surveys. *International journal for equity in health*, *13*(1), 18.https://equityhealthj.biomedcentral.com/articles/10.1186/1475-9276-13-18

Harrison, J. S., Freeman, R. E., & Sá de Abreu, M. C. (2015). Stakeholder theory as an ethical approach to effective management: Applying the theory to multiple contexts. *Revista Brasileira De Gestão De Negócios*, *17*858-859. doi:10.7819/rbgn.v17i55.2647

Harrison, J. S., & Wicks, A. C. (2013). Stakeholder theory, value, and firm performance. *Business ethics quarterly*, *23*(1), 97-124.

Hasnas, J. (2013). Whither stakeholder theory? A guide for the perplexed revisited. *Journal of Business Ethics, 112*(1), 47-57. doi:10.1007/s10551-012-1231-8

Houghton, C., Casey, D., Shaw, D., & Murphy, K. (2013). Rigor in qualitative case-study research. *Nurse Researcher, 20*(4), 12-17. Retrieved from https://doi.org/10.7748/nr2013.03.20.4.12.e326

Hechanova, M. R. M., Melgar, I., Falguera, P. Z., & Villaverde, M. (2014). Organisational culture and workplace corruption in government hospitals. *Journal of Pacific Rim Psychology, 8*(2), 62-70. doi.org/10.1017/prp.2014.5

Heravi, A., Coffey, V., & Trigunarsyah, B. (2015). Evaluating the level of stakeholder involvement during the project planning processes of building projects. *International Journal of Project Management, 33*985-997. doi:10.1016/j.ijproman.2014.12.007

154

Hope, K. R. (2014). Kenya's corruption problem: causes and consequences. *Commonwealth & Comparative Politics, 52*(4), 493-512. doi:10.1080/14662043.2014.955981

Hofstede. G. & Hofstede, G.J. (2005). *Cultures and Organizations. Software of the Mind* (2nd Ed.). New York, NY: McGraw-Hill.

Hühn, M. P., & Dierksmeier, C. (2016). Will the real A. Smith please stand up! *Journal of Business Ethics, 136*(1), 119-132. doi:10.1007/s10551-014-2506-z

Jakubowski, A., Stearns, S. C., Kruk, M. E., Angeles, G., & Thirumurthy, H. (2017). The US President's malaria initiative and under-5 child mortality in sub-Saharan Africa: A difference-in-differences analysis. *Plos Medicine, 14*(6), 1-20. doi:10.1371/journal.pmed.1002319

Kagotho, N., Bunger, A., & Wagner, K. (2016). "They make money off of us" a phenomenological analysis of consumer perceptions of corruption in Kenya's HIV response system. *BMC Health Services Research, 161*-11.doi:10.1186/s12913-016-1721

Kankeu, H. T., Boyer, S., Fodjo Toukam, R., & Abu-Zaineh, M. (2016). How do supply-side factors influence informal payments for healthcare? The case of HIV patients in Cameroon. *The International Journal of Health Planning and Management, 31*(1), E41-E57. doi:10.1002/hpm.2266

Kankeu, H. T., & Ventelou, B. (2016). Socioeconomic inequalities in informal payments for health care: An assessment of the 'Robin Hood' hypothesis in 33 African countries. *Social Science & Medicine, 151*173-186. doi:10.1016/j.socscimed.2016.01.015

Kvale, S. (2008). *Doing interviews.* Thousand Oaks, CA: Sage.

Kvale, S. (1996). *Interviews: An introduction to qualitative research interviewing.* Thousand Oaks, CA: Sage.

Liu, X. (2016). Corruption culture and corporate misconduct. *Journal of Financial Economics, 122*(2), 307-327. doi.10.1016/j.jfineco.2016.06.005

Lewellyn, K. B., & Bao, S. (2017). The role of national culture and corruption on managing earnings around the world. *Journal of World Business, 52*798-808. doi:10.1016/j.jwb.2017.07.002

Lucae, S., Rebentisch, E. R., & Oehmen, J. (2014). Understanding the front-end of largescale engineering programs. *Procedia Computer Science, 28*(1), 653-662. doi:10.1016/j.procs.2014.03.079

Luiz, J., & Stewart, C. (2014). Corruption, South African multinational enterprises and institutions in Africa. *Journal of Business Ethics, 124*(3), 383-398. doi:10.1007/s10551-013-1878-9

Mbuagbaw, L., Thabane, L., Ongolo-Zogo, P., & Lang, T. (2011). The challenges and opportunities of conducting a clinical trial in a low resource setting: the case of the Cameroon mobile phone SMS (CAMPS) trial, an investigator initiated trial. *Trials, 12*(1), 145. doi: 10.1186/1745-6215-12-145

Magill, M., Quinzii, M., & Rochet, J. C. (2015). A theory of the stakeholder corporation. *Econometrica, 83*(5), 1685-1725. doi:10.3982/ECTA11455

Markham, W. T., & Fonjong, L. (2015). Geography, demography, and environmental problems. In *Saving the Environment in Sub-Saharan Africa* (pp. 49-60). Palgrave Macmillan US. doi:10.1057/9781137507198_4

Mason, C., & Simmons, J. (2014). Embedding corporate social responsibility in corporate governance: A stakeholder systems approach. *Journal of Business Ethics, 119*(1), 77-86. doi:10.1007/s10551-012-1615-9

Mattingly, J. 2004. Stakeholder salience, structural development, and firm performance: Structural and performance correlates of sociopolitical stakeholder management strategies. *Business and Society,* 43(1): 97-114. http://dx.doi.org/10.1177/0007650304263415

McManus, J., & Webley, S. (2013, Spring). An ethical perspective of stakeholder salience. *Management Services Journal, 57*(2), 32–36. Retrieved from http://www.ims productivity.com/page.cfm/content/Management-Services-Journal/

Mengistu, B., Hassan, S., & Teklu, T. (2013). Public perceptions of corruption in Ethiopia: Assessment and descriptive analysis. *International Journal of Business & Public Administration,* 10(2), 90. doi:10.1080/17475759.2011.558317

Miles, S. (2017). Stakeholder theory classification: a theoretical and empirical evaluation of definitions. *Journal of Business Ethics, 142*(3), 437-459.doi.org/10.1007/s10551-015 2741-y

Mimba, N. H., Helden, G. J., & Tillema, S. (2013). The design and use of performance Information in Indonesian local governments under diverging stakeholder pressures. Public Administration & Development, 33(1), 15. doi:10.1002/pad.1612

Michele J., M., & Janice M., M. (2015). Situating and constructing diversity in semi-structured interviews. *Global Qualitative Nursing Research, 2,* 1-12. doi:10.1177/2333393615597674

Molem-Christopher, S., Beri-Parfait, B., & Ntangsi-Max, M. (2017). Determinants of the inefficiency of public hospitals in Cameroon. *International Journal of Academic Research in Business and Social Sciences, 7*(6), 404-419. doi:10.6007/IJARBSS/v7 i6/2998

Montoya, A., Calvert, C., & Filippi, V. (2014). Explaining differences in maternal mortality levels in sub-Saharan African hospitals: a systematic review and meta-analysis. *International health, 6*(1), 12-22. doi.org/10.1093/inthealth/iht037

Mostert, S., Njuguna, F., Olbara, G., Sindano, S., Sitaresmi, M. N., Supriyadi, E., & Kaspers, G.

(2015). Series: Corruption in health-care systems and its effect on cancer care in Africa. *The Lancet Oncology, 16,* e394–e404. https://doi-org.proxy1.ncu.edu/10.1016/S1470-2045(15)00163-1

Nana, G. (2016). Language Ideology and the Colonial Legacy in Cameroon Schools: A Historical Perspective. *Journal of Education and Training Studies, 4*(4), 168-196. doi: https://doi.org/10.11114/jets.v4i4.1385

Nguemegne, J. P. (2011). Fighting corruption in Africa: The anti-corruption system in Cameroon. *International Journal of Organization Theory and Behavior, 14*(1), 83-121.Retrieved from http://search.proquest.com.proxy1.ncu.edu/docview/8674 21978?accountid=28180

Njong, A., & Ngantcha, J. (2013). Institutions and leakage of public funds in the Cameroonian healthcare delivery chain. *Journal of African Development, 15*(1), 19-43. Retrieved from http://www.jadafea.com/wpcontent/uploads/2014/07/J AD_vol15_ch2.pdf

Noland, J., & Phillips, R. (2010). Stakeholder engagement, discourse ethics and strategic management. *International Journal of Management Reviews, 12*(1), 39-49. doi:10.1111/j.1468-2370.2009.00279.x

Norman, W. (2015). Rawls on markets and corporate governance. *Business Ethics Quarterly, 25*(1), 29-64. doi:10.1017/beq.2015.16

Ongolo-Zogo, P., Lavis, J. N., Tomson, G., & Sewankambo, N. K. (2014). Initiatives supporting evidence informed health system policymaking in Cameroon and Uganda: a comparative historical case study. *BMC Health Services Research, 14*612. doi:10.1186/s12913-014-0612-3

Osifo, O. C. (2014). An ethical governance perspective on anti-corruption policies and procedures: Agencies and trust in Cameroon, Ghana, and Nigeria evaluation. *International Journal of Public Administration, 37*(5), 308-327.

http://dx.doi.org.proxy1.ncu.edu/10.1080/01900692.2013.
836663

Osifo, O. C. (2014). An ethical governance perspective on anti-corruption policies and procedures: Agencies and trust in Cameroon, Ghana, and Nigeria evaluation. *International Journal of Public Administration, 37*(5), 308-327.
http://dx.doi.org.proxy1.ncu.edu/10.1080/01900692.2013.
836663

Owoye, O., & Bissessar, N. (2014). Corruption in African countries: A symptom of leadership and institutional failure. In *Challenges to democratic governance in developing countries* (pp. 227-245). Springer International Publishing.

Pellegrini, L., & Gerlagh, R. (2008). Causes of corruption: a survey of cross-country analyses and extended results. *Economics of Governance, 9*(3), 245-263. doi:10.1007/s10101-007 0033-4

Pena-López, J., & Sánchez Santos, J. (2014). Does corruption have social roots? The role of culture and social capital. *Journal of Business Ethics, 122*(4), 697-708.
doi:10.1007/s10551-013-1789-9

Pillay, S., & Kluvers, R. (2014). An institutional theory perspective on corruption: The case of a developing democracy. *Financial Accountability & Management, 30*(1), 95-119. doi:10.1111/faam.12029

Pillay, P. (2017). Anti-Corruption agencies in South Africa and Brazil: trends and challenges. *African Journal of Public Affairs, 9*(8), 1-14.

Popescu, L. (2013). From a holistic approach of public policy to co-governance. *Theoretical & Applied Economics, 20*(7), 95-108. Retrieved from http:// www.
econpapers.repec.org/article/agrjournl/v_3axx_3ay_3a201
3_3ai_3a7

Poppo, L., & Zhou, K. Z. (2014). Managing contracts for fairness in buyer–supplier exchanges. *Strategic Management Journal, 35*(10), 1508-1527. doi:10.1002/smj.2175

Purnell, L. S., & Freeman, R. E. (2012). Stakeholder theory, fact/value dichotomy, and the normative core: How Wall Street stops the ethics conversation. *Journal of Business Ethics, 109*(1), 109–116. http://dx.doi.org/10.1007/s10551-012-1383-6

Quah, J. T. (2016). Combating corruption in six Asian countries: a comparative analysis. *Asian Education & Development Studies, 5*(2), 244. doi:10.1108/AEDS-01-2016-0011

Robinson, O. C. (2014). Sampling in interview-based qualitative research: A theoretical and practical guide. *Qualitative Research in Psychology, 11*(1), 25-41 doi.org/10.1080/14780887.2013.801543

Sabella, A., Kashou, R., & Omran, O. (2014). Quality management practices and their relationship to organizational performance. *International Journal of Operations & Production Management, 34*(12), 1487-1505. doi/abs/10.1108/IJOPM-04-2013-0210

Safadi, N. S., & Lombe, M. (2013). Exploring factors associated with citizens' perception of a country's economic condition: The case of Palestine. *Social Development Issues, 35*(1), 43-54. doi:10.1016/j.forpol.2015.08.004.

Salomon, J. A., Wang, H., Freeman, M. K., Vos, T., Flaxman, A. D., Lopez, A. D., & Murray, C. J. (2013). Healthy life expectancy for 187 countries, 1990–2010: a systematic analysis for the Global Burden Disease Study 2010. *The Lancet, 380*(9859), 2144-2162. doi: 10.1016/S0140-6736(12)61690-0

Savage, G., Nix, T., Whitehead, J., & Blair, J. (1991). Strategies for assessing and managing organizational stakeholders. *Academy of Management Review, 5*(2), 61–75. doi:10.5465/AME.1991.4274682

Smith, A. (1776). *The Wealth of Nations*. Glasgow, Scotland: Strahan and Cadell

Søreide, T., & Truex, R. (2013). Multi-stakeholder groups for better sector performance: A key to fighting corruption in natural-resource governance? *Development Policy Review, 31*(2), 203. doi:10.1111/dpr.12003

Stake, R. E. (1996). *The Art of Case Study Research*. Thousand Oaks, CA: Sage Publications, Inc.

Stamati, T., Papadopoulos, T., & Anagnostopoulos, D. (2015). Social media for openness and accountability in the public sector: Cases in the Greek context. Government Information Quarterly, 3 (2), 3212-3229. doi:10.1016/j.giq.2014.11.004

Starks, H., Shaw, J. L., Hiratsuka, V., Dillard, D. A., & Robinson, R. (2015). Engaging stakeholders to develop a depression management decision support tool in a tribal health system. *Quality of Life Research, 24*(5), 1097-1105. doi:10.1007/s11136-014-0810-9

Stone, B. (2015). Accountability and the design of an anticorruption agency in a parliamentary democracy. *Policy Studies, 36*(2), 157-175. doi:10.1080/01442872.2014.1000844

Stuart, H. C., & Moore, C. (2017). Shady characters: The implications of illicit organizational roles for resilient team performance. *Academy of Management Journal, 60*(5), 1963 1985. doi:10.5465/amj.2014.0512

Tantalo, C. and Priem, R.L. (2014). Value creation through stakeholder synergy. *Strategic Management Journal*, doi: 10.1002/smj.2337.

Tashman, P., & Raelin, J. (2013). Who and what really matters to the firm: Moving stakeholder salience beyond managerial perceptions. *Business Ethics Quarterly, 23*(4), 591-616. doi:10.5840/beq201323441

Tinyami Erick, T., YongMin, C., Akam, A. J., Afoh, C. O., Seung Hun, R., Min Seok, C., & Jae Wook, C. (2015). Cameroon

161

public health sector: shortage and inequalities in geographic distribution of health personnel. *International Journal for Equity in Health*, *14*(1), 1-12. doi:10.1186/s12939-015-0172-0

Tormusa, D. O., & Idom, A. M. (2016). The impediments of corruption on the efficiency of healthcare service delivery in Nigeria. *Online Journal of Health Ethics*, *12*(1), 10-21. doi:10.18785/ojhe.1201.03

Treisman, D. (2007). What have we learned about the causes of corruption from ten years of cross-national empirical research? *Annual Review of Political Science*, 10:211-244. Retrieved from https://doi.org/10.1146/annurev.polisci.10.081205.095418

Walton, G. W., & Peiffer, C. (2017). The impacts of education and institutional trust on citizens' willingness to report corruption: lessons from Papua New Guinea. *Australian Journal of Political Science*, *52*(4), 517-536. doi:10.1080/10361146.2017.1374346

Yamb, B., & Bayemi, O. (2016). Bribery in Cameroonian public hospitals: Who pays who and how much? *Asian journal of Social Sciences and Management Studies*, *3*(1), 7-17. Retrieved from https://ideas.repec.org/a/aoj/ajssms/2016p7-17.html

Yamb, B., & Bayemi, O. (2017). Corruption forms and heath care provision in Douala metropolis public hospitals of Cameroon. *Turkish Economic Review*, *4*(1), 96105. doi:http://dx.doi.org.proxy1.ncu.edu/10.1453/ter.v4i1.1206

Yang, R. J., Yaowu, W., & Xiao-Hua, J. (2014). Stakeholders' attributes, behaviors, and decision-making strategies in construction projects: Importance and correlations in practice. *Project Management Journal*, *45*(3), 74-90. doi:10.1002/pmj.21412

Yang, R. J., Zou, P. X., & Wang, J. (2016). Modelling stakeholder-associated risk networks in green building projects. International Journal of Project Management, 3(4), 3466-3481. doi:10.1016/j.ijproman.2015.09.010

Yin, R. K. (2009). *Case study research*: Design and methods. Thousand Oaks, CA: Sage Publications, Inc.

Yin, R. K. (2013a). *Qualitative research from start to finish*. New York, NY: The Guilford Press.

Yin, R. K. (2013b). Validity and generalization in future case study evaluations. Evaluation: *The International Journal of Theory, Research and Practice, 19*(3), 321-332. doi:10.1177/1356389013497081

Zhong, N., Wang, S., & Yang, R. (2017). Does corporate governance enhance common interests of shareholders and primary stakeholders? *Journal of Business Ethics, 141*(2), 411-431.doi10.1007%2Fs10551-016-3347-8

Printed in the United States
By Bookmasters